NURSING ETHICS

Nursing Ethics

A Principle-Based Approach

2nd Edition

Steven D. Edwards

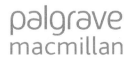

palgrave
macmillan

First edition 1996
Reprinted eleven times
Second edition 2009

Published by
PALGRAVE MACMILLAN

Palgrave Macmillan in the UK is an imprint of Macmillan Publishers Limited, registered in England, company number 785998, of Houndmills, Basingstoke, Hampshire RG21 6XS.

Palgrave Macmillan in the US is a division of St Martin's Press LLC, 175 Fifth Avenue, New York, NY 10010.

Palgrave Macmillan is the global academic imprint of the above companies and has companies and representatives throughout the world.

Palgrave® and Macmillan® are registered trademarks in the United States, the United Kingdom, Europe and other countries

ISBN-13: 978-0-230-20590-1
ISBN-10: 0-230-20590-9

This book is printed on paper suitable for recycling and made from fully managed and sustained forest sources. Logging, pulping and manufacturing processes are expected to conform to the environmental regulations of the country of origin.

A catalogue record for this book is available from the British Library.

A catalog record for this book is available from the Library of Congress.

10 9 8 7 6 5 4 3 2 1
18 17 16 15 14 13 12 11 10 09

Printed in China

Contents

Preface   vii

Introduction   ix

1   Preliminary Matters   1
    What is ethics?   1
    Why should nurses study ethics?   6
    The inherent moral dimension of nursing practice   9
    How can moral issues be identified?   12
    Conclusion   17

2   Judgements, Rules, Principles and Theories   18
    Moral judgements   19
    Moral rules   20
    Moral principles   26
    Moral theories: utilitarianism, deontology, virtue theory   29
    How are the four levels related?   47
    Arguments for the priority of moral principles   49
    Conclusion   55

3   The Four Principles: Respect for Autonomy, Beneficence, Non-maleficence and Justice   56
    The principle of respect for autonomy   57
    The principle of beneficence   74
    The principle of non-maleficence   80
    The principle of justice   86
    Respect for autonomy as the weightiest principle?   98
    The principles and the NMC Code (2008)   101
    Conclusion   105

4 **Conflicts between the Principles**   106
 Respect for autonomy in conflict with beneficence
  and non-maleficence   106
 Autonomy in conflict with justice: allocation of
  scarce resources   127
 Conclusion   146

5 **Care-Based Ethics: A Challenge to the
 Principle-Based Approach?**   147
 Clouser and Gert's critique   148
 A care-based approach: the first wave   149
 The second wave   169
 The third wave   174
 'Principles infused with care' approach   176
 Conclusion   180

6 **Applying the 'Principles Infused with Care'
 Approach in the Context of Genetics**   182
 Case one: Prenatal screening for Down's syndrome   184
 Case two: A request to keep genetic
  information confidential   196
 Case three: A decision to have radical surgery
  on the basis of genetic information   200
 Conclusion   202

7 **Supererogatory Actions in the Context of Nursing**   203
 What are supererogatory acts?   205
 To whom do nurses have obligations?   207
 Do nurses undertake supererogatory acts?
  Five nurse case examples   211
 Conclusion   220

Appendix: NMC Code of Conduct (2008)   221

Bibliography   228

Index   237

Preface

I have tried to produce a degree-level text in nursing ethics, but one which will be of use to nursing diploma students, to those studying nursing ethics at postgraduate level and to registered nurses who are undertaking short courses in nursing ethics. I became aware of the need for such a text between 1991 and 1993. During this period I was required to write and to teach a number of courses in nursing ethics at varying levels. There are, of course, several books on nursing ethics, but none seemed to be at just the right level for the needs of the students I taught. Although many students found Melia (1989) and Chadwick and Tadd (1992) extremely useful introductions to the subject, these texts seemed not to provide material beyond diploma level.

The most thorough treatment of health care ethics that I am aware of is Beauchamp and Childress's Principles of Biomedical Ethics (1989, 1994). It is no understatement to reveal that this book changed my whole outlook on nursing ethics and this is evident throughout the following text. The students I taught, however, did not seem to find Beauchamp and Childress user-friendly; they found it too dense and too medically orientated. Hence, it has been my intention to provide a text which approximates the systematicity of Beauchamp and Childress's work, but which is more accessible to students of nursing ethics.

When I trained as a nurse, the curriculum included no ethics whatsoever. Yet, the moral problems encountered during my time in nursing drove me to study philosophy at undergraduate level. It soon became apparent that, at that time (the mid-eighties), the subject matter of ethics courses made no mention of the kinds of moral problems which arise in nursing practice. Further, I came to realise that the problem of moral knowledge was merely a part of a larger problem of knowledge in general. This led me into the problem of philosophical relativism and far away from applied ethics.

A peculiar chain of events resulted in my obtaining a post which involved nothing other than teaching nursing ethics. This gave me the opportunity to re-examine the moral problems which I had faced as a nurse many years earlier, and this book forms part of that ongoing examination.

I have benefited greatly over the years from discussion of moral matters with very many people. But I would like to acknowledge particular debts of gratitude to the 1991 intake of nursing students at Buckinghamshire College of Higher Education, to ED Lepper and to Simon Woods.

STEVEN D. EDWARDS
Swansea 1996

Introduction

As was the first edition, this book is an attempt to apply to nursing ethics the approach to bioethics, which is set out by Beauchamp and Childress in their *Principles of Biomedical Ethics* (2009). It should be stressed at the outset, though, that there are differences between the claims set out by Beauchamp and Childress and claims made in this book. Further, one of these differences is quite fundamental in that in their book they explicitly reject any hierarchical ordering of principles (2009, p. viii), but in the present text it is tentatively claimed that the principle of respect for autonomy is 'weightier', so to speak, than other moral principles.

No attempt has been made to discuss or describe all the types of moral problems which nurses are likely to encounter during the course of their practice; any such attempt is doomed to failure. Instead, what has been done is to try to set out a general approach which can then be applied to very many of the types of moral problems which arise in nursing practice. In particular, the approach set out here applies to moral problems arising from attempts to care for competent patients, though attention is also given to situations in which patients are unable to make decisions for themselves.

Chapter 1 begins with an attempt to offer an outline of some of the ways in which people understand the term 'ethics'; this is followed by arguments in support of the claim that nurses should study ethics, and the outline of a strategy to aid recognition of moral issues. In addition, a discussion has been included of the concepts of moral awareness, perception and imagination. This is added to try to say more about the experience of noticing and responding to the ethical dimension of nursing practice.

Chapter 2 describes four levels of thought about moral matters: judgements, rules, principles and theories. It is argued that, of these, it is moral principles which provide the most helpful tools for the analysis and response to moral problems in nursing.

Due to the conclusion drawn from Chapter 2, Chapter 3 consists in a description of each of the four principles, whilst Chapter 4 focuses on the application of them. It is proposed that the onus of justification lies with those who attempt to override the competent, autonomous decisions of patients. As will be evident to readers, the application of this position to the moral problems arising from the care of persons with suicidal intentions causes great problems and the position arrived at is, it seems, supported by reason but conflicts with the emotions. This very conflict takes us to the heart of a challenge to the principle-based approach from the perspective of a care-based approach to ethics. Chapter 5 tries to address the challenge. It is argued that the principle-based approach defended here can resist such criticisms, although the approach defended incorporates one idea of care taken from Nel Noddings's work (1984). Nonetheless, the approach which is developed here is still a principle-based approach, albeit one which is 'infused with care'.

In Chapter 5, following a brief summary of the kinds of ethical issues raised by developments in genetics, we focus on three specific cases. These involve, respectively: a decision to terminate a foetus diagnosed with Down's syndrome, a problem regarding a request to a nurse that she keeps confidential information regarding a patient's hereditary disease, and lastly a problem regarding a decision to have radical surgery based upon receipt of genetic information. In the analysis of the first case, in particular, a lengthy illustration is given of the way in which the principle-based approach defended here can be applied to a real situation.

The concluding chapter of the book is perhaps the most abstract. It attempts to show how the principles operant in the principle-based approach can help to structure thought concerning matters within nursing ethics, and to foster clearer analysis and thinking in relation to such matters. As is explained in the chapter, the nursing context has changed in such a way since the time of writing the first edition that some of the rationale for including a discussion of supererogation has been undermined. However, with the help of case examples, it is shown that nurses cannot routinely be expected to perform supererogatory acts.

Overall, it is fair to say that most of the book has been re-written and updated. And, as has just been mentioned, there is a completely new chapter on ethical issues in genetics. Moreover, during the period in which this edition was being prepared the NMC produced a new code (NMC, 2008), and Beauchamp and Childress produced a 6th edition of their book (Beauchamp and Childress, 2009). The present text has been updated to incorporate these important recent publications.

Lastly, I would like to express thanks to colleagues who have helped me with the preparation of this book, in particular Hugh Upton, Mike McNamee, Thomas Schramme, Susanne Darra, Jeanette Hewitt and Nic Bowler. Thanks are due also to four anonymous referees who provided helpful comments on an earlier draft of the text.

STEVEN EDWARDS
Swansea 2009

Chapter 1

Preliminary Matters

This chapter begins by offering a definition of ethics, and highlighting three different senses of it. Then it is explained why it is important for nurses to think about, discuss and study ethics. Then, following introduction of the ideas of moral awareness, perception and imagination, a strategy to develop sensitivity to the moral dimension of nursing practice is presented.

What is ethics?

Consider these four examples of ethical issues, three of which are being widely discussed at the time of writing (May 2008).

The first one concerns so-called 'mixed sex' wards (BBC, 19/5/08, 'Mixed-sex NHS still a problem'). This news item refers to the distress and embarrassment which many people feel when they are patients in a mixed-sex ward. It makes plain that patients should not need to walk past patients of the opposite sex when they are going for a wash or to use the toilet. Many patients strongly dislike being cared for in such circumstances. At a vulnerable time in their lives, it seems, they are subjected to yet further humiliation.

The second item concerns midwifery services in South East Wales. Concern has been expressed about the standards of maternity provision in two hospitals in the region. It is reported that due to low staffing levels, it has not been possible to provide a safe service for mothers-to-be. As a result, an enquiry has taken place and happily the situation looks now to be on the way to being improved. The concerns about poor levels of care in the region were expressed by the Royal College of Midwives (RCM) (BBC, 20/5/08, 'Urgent action on maternity units').

The third item involves abortion. Last night (20/5/08) MPs in the UK had the option of voting to lower the current limits within which an abortion can legally take place. The current upper limit is 24 weeks. Some MPs thought that should be lowered to 20 weeks because advancements in medical science now make it possible for some very premature babies to survive, even though they are born before 24 weeks. Thus, some argued, because babies are 'viable' below 24 week gestation, then abortions at 24 weeks should not be legally permitted.

The fourth example of an ethical issue to be described briefly now, is not one which will feature in any newspaper headline. Suppose you are working as a nurse. You are giving a patient his or her medication. You place the tablets in the plastic container in his or her hand, and you have checked he or she has a glass of water within their reach. In your previous interactions with this patient he has seemed quite cheerful. But now he looks anxious. You ask him if everything is ok? Is there anything on his mind? Does he need some help?

This isn't the kind of episode of care which will make a news story, but it is an ethical issue. You show your concern about the patient by, first of all, *noticing* that all might not be well with him, and by responding to this.

These are four descriptions of situations which raise ethical issues. They are situations with an ethical dimension, as we will say here. In the first example, patients feel distressed at having to be cared for in a mixed-sex ward. In the second, there are risks of harm to pregnant mothers and their babies. In the third, there are disagreements about how to balance a woman's rights over her own body against the right to life of the foetus. And in the last example, a nurse notices and responds to her suspicion that a patient is worried about something. All the situations involve various kinds of harms and benefits to those involved and this indicates that they are situations with an ethical dimension to them.

Shortly, we will attempt to describe how situations with an ethical dimension can be identified more systematically. But before this it will prove useful to set out a rough distinction between three senses of the term 'ethics': personal ethics, group ethics, and philosophical ethics. For present purposes, we can follow the convention of regarding the terms 'ethics' and 'morals' as synonyms (Singer, 1979, p. 1, 1991, p. v; Seedhouse, 1988, p. 18).

Personal ethics

The first sense of the term 'ethics' to be mentioned here concerns its use in the personal sense. When invited to offer a definition of ethics, many people understand the term in this fashion. Ethics in the personal sense, they suggest, refers to the beliefs which individuals hold about ethical issues. Such beliefs stem from the informal moral education received from various sources: parents, schoolteachers, religious figures and the media. These sources influence the views of people about moral matters and typically inform the intuitive responses people offer about ethical issues.

Most of us have opinions on ethical issues whether or not we have formally studied ethics. Someone may claim that it is wrong to abuse children or to kill animals for sport, for example. Such personal beliefs may be the result of deliberation by the persons concerned, in which case it could be expected that they are able to supply reasons in support of their views. They may argue, for example, that it is wrong to kill animals for sport because it is wrong to kill humans for sport, and humans are animals. A person who argues against killing animals in this way may assume there to be no significant distinction in morality between killing humans and killing non-human animals.

Alternatively, a person might not be able to provide any reasons in support of his or her view; such a person may say simply that he or she knows it is wrong to kill animals for sport without being able to say just why it is wrong. In everyday arguments about moral issues, people frequently appeal to their moral intuitions: they claim simply to know that some courses of action are wrong even though they cannot say why. Child abuse presents a useful example here. Most of us find this practice morally abhorrent, and, generally, do not believe that any reasons are required in support of such a view: 'it is wrong to abuse children and that's that' we think.

Almost all people, able to express a view, hold positions on many situations with an ethical dimension. These positions reflect their own ethics: their own views of what is right and what is wrong. Let us turn now to look at 'group ethics'.

Group ethics

A second sense of the term 'ethics', of particular relevance to nurses, involves reference to the ethics of a group. These may be formal statements of standards of behaviour which members are expected to act in accordance with. Such a group might be a professional group such as nurses, footballers or medical staff, or a religious group – we could think of the Ten Commandments in this context.

Nurses comprise a useful example of a professional group which has proposed various codes of ethics. For example, the American Nurses Association (ANA) has set out a Code of Ethics which identifies the standards of behaviour expected of its members (see Benjamin and Curtis, 1986, pp. 179–81). The equivalent bodies in the UK, the United Kingdom Central Council for Nursing, Midwifery and Health Visiting (UKCC) and the Nursing and Midwifery Council (NMC) have set out Codes of Conduct which perform a similar function (UKCC, 1992; NMC, 2008). Since there is a plethora of literature concerning codes of conduct for nurses, this second sense of the term 'ethics' will not be pursued for now. (For further information on codes of conduct, see Burnard and Chapman, 1988; Chadwick and Tadd, 1992; Thompson, Melia and Boyd, 2000.)

Philosophical ethics

The third, and last, sense of the term 'ethics' to be identified here refers to ethics as a more formal, academic enterprise, which we can usefully describe as philosophical ethics. Within this, we can distinguish three general types of activity.

1. The development of *ethical theories* which attempt to set out prescriptions for morally right action. This may be done by attempting to show that acts which accord with certain specified criteria are morally right and others morally wrong. Such criteria comprise a set of justifications for particular actions, or types of actions. Hence, a particular act, A (say, telling the truth), may be judged to be morally obligatory since A accords with the criteria proposed in the theory. Two examples of theories devised in this way are Utilitarianism (Mill, 1863) and Kant's duty-based moral theory (Kant, 1785). Crudely, according to the Utilitarian, acts are right in so far as they maximize benefits or minimize harms. And, equally crudely, according to Kant,

the rightness or wrongness of an act depends upon the motives of the actor.

We will be looking at these two moral theories, together with virtue theory, in greater detail in the next chapter. They are given here as examples of one of the kinds of activities which fall within philosophical ethics. It should be added that the approach to ethics to be set out in this book may amount to a theory in the sense under discussion here, for, as will be seen, the approach attempts to identify justifications for acting in one way rather than in others.

2. A second component of philosophical ethics consists in the *analytical enterprise* of examining moral claims, concepts and theories. This involves, for example, searching for inconsistency in moral argument and lack of clarity in moral concepts. This enterprise differs from the first activity discussed above in that it does not itself involve the proposal of substantive claims concerning what constitutes right or wrong action.

We will be required to engage in philosophical ethics in this second sense. As will be seen, it is important to be especially clear when it comes to definitions of key terms and principles. Attention to clarity reduces the risk of misunderstanding and fosters a rigorous approach to the subject matter.

3. The third kind of activity describable under the rubric of philosophical ethics is so-called *metaethics*. This involves an examination of the language of morals itself. From the perspective of metaethics one asks questions such as: Can there be any moral facts? Is moral language meaningful? This differs from the second type of philosophical ethics in the sense that it queries the whole nature and language of morals.

We will not be engaged in any metaethical tasks in this book. It will simply be presumed – not unreasonably – that moral language is meaningful. Nor will the question of whether there can be moral facts be addressed (those interested may find Raphael [1981] a useful introduction). It is not being presumed that there are such facts, rather, it is supposed here that that question is less relevant to our concerns than the matters to be investigated during the course of this book.

This, then, completes a description of three senses of the term 'ethics'. Before moving on to the next section, it is worth pausing briefly to consider the relations between these three kinds of activity, and also to consider their relevance to members of the nursing profession. It is clear that the majority of nurses hold ethical views; hence they have an ethics in the first sense of the term described above. It is also clear that these beliefs about moral matters which individual nurses hold carry implications for the way certain moral problems encountered in professional practice will be viewed. For example, nurses who believe homosexual relationships to be morally wrong may find it difficult to deal with patients who are homosexual.

Furthermore, a nurse who believes homosexual activities to be morally wrong, might find that this particular moral view conflicts with certain clauses in the NMC Code, for example, 'You must not discriminate in any way against those in your care' (NMC, 2008; see Appendix). If the nurse found she could not care for patients who are homosexual she would then experience a conflict between her personal ethics, which inclines her to avoid homosexual patients, and the stand-ards of behaviour required by the NMC Code. Thus there is a conflict between the personal ethics of the nurse and the 'group ethics' of the professional group to whom she belongs. This is so, of course, because the NMC Code is compiled largely by members of the nursing profes-sion. It is evident, then, that courses of action which accord with one's personal ethical beliefs can conflict with courses of action required by the code recommended by one's professional body.

Engaging in some philosophical ethics can help to expose the source of such conflicts; this can be done by analysing and making explicit the moral principles which clash in such situations. We spend some time doing this in the explication of the four principles in chapter four below. Hopefully, the reader will be better equipped to undertake such analyses of moral conflicts after reading this book. For now, we move on to consider just why nurses should study ethics.

Why should nurses study ethics?

Ethical problems are faced continuously in our day-to-day lives. Suppose you are walking down a city centre street, a person who looks unwell, and painfully thin asks you for money for food. Should you give him or her some? The situation has an ethical dimension to it since you are in a position to benefit the person by giving them some money; and you might be said to cause harm, if only indirectly, if you walk by without helping the person.

Take another example. You notice an appeal in a newspaper which points out that a donation of £250 can save someone's sight, maintain the life of a person in an extremely poor country (if only for a month or two) or fund an operation to repair a cleft palate. Should you send a donation? There are countless other, more mundane, examples of moral problems encountered on a regular basis: Should you tell your friend the horrible truth about his new haircut? Should you try to avoid paying the bill at a restaurant? Should you 'jump the queue' at the supermarket checkout because you are in a hurry? Clearly, we are capable of arriving at decisions concerning moral matters and can do so without doing a course in ethics. So why should nurses study ethics?

Below are some reasons which are relevant, and which help to support the claim that the moral intuition acquired and relied upon in ordinary, everyday circumstances is of limited use in the health care setting (Hussey, 1990).

- First, it is true to say that as a nurse one is faced with many more ethical problems than most ordinary members of the community have to face. In some kinds of occupations it is possible to drift along happily without ever facing a serious moral dilemma. The sheer quantity of moral problems faced in the health care setting differs greatly from the quantity of moral problems one faces, generally speaking, in ordinary life. So, the moral context within which every day moral intuition is developed differs from the health care setting at least in the respect that in nursing practice the number of moral problems faced by nurses is significantly greater than is encountered by many people in many other types of occupations.

- Second, in our normal dealings with people on a day-to-day basis, we find people in their normal state – at home, at work, or in the shops etc. They are in familiar surroundings with people they know, and typically they are in a situation in which they feel comfortable. Clearly, none of this is true when patients are in hospital or when they or their close relatives are seriously ill. Patients may be anxious, feel insecure, or perhaps be unconscious. So the usual, conventional setting within which we make moral decisions can again be seen to be radically different from the health care setting.

- Third, it may be the case that as a nurse one comes into contact with people who have had a different kind of moral education, and so have developed different ways of responding to moral problems – they have a personal ethics which differs radically from one's own. Consider, here, people from different ethnic backgrounds or people with different religious or political views. Many people do not have any prolonged contact with others who have had a radically different moral education than themselves. So, again, it can be seen that moral decision-making in nursing practice may differ from moral decision-making in ordinary circumstances. This is so because the nurse needs to take into account the perspective of the person who has a different moral outlook than he or she. The nurse is, in fact, required to do this by the NMC (2008).

In ordinary, everyday life some people consider their own moral intuition to be unfailingly correct. For such people, moral conflicts do not arise. They simply assume that any moral views which diverge from the ones they themselves endorse must be wrong. But such an attitude is unsupportable. It is necessary to consider at least the possibility that other moral views may be correct before it is possible to make any kind of adjudication between conflicting moral claims. It is not enough just to assert one's own moral views without considering other perspectives, and it is especially important for health care professionals to recognize this.

- Fourth, the availability of complex medical technology and advances in sciences such as genetics again makes the situation in the health care setting radically different from the normal context within which moral decisions are made. In the health care setting the nurse will encounter moral dilemmas of a type which he or she will not have encountered previously in ordinary everyday life. These might be very dramatic, such as end of life decisions, or less dramatic but still of vital importance, for example how to deal with a patient who feels anxious and vulnerable due to their health problem. Again, these points reinforce the view that the moral intuition developed in ordinary life is unlikely to be adequate to cope with the complex moral problems which arise in the health care context.

These last four points seem enough to support the claim that nurses should study ethics. It does seem plausible that the moral intuition developed and relied upon in normal circumstances may be inadequate to cope with the quantity and the complexity of moral issues encountered in the health care setting. But there is an even stronger reason why it is important to learn about ethics and to develop a capacity to respond in the right way to ethical problems in practice. This stems from the inherent ethical dimension of such practice.

The inherent moral dimension of nursing practice

There is an inescapable ethical dimension to nursing practice. Every action undertaken by a nurse in the course of that practice has an ethical dimension to it. This is because nursing acts are directed towards moral ends. They aim to bring about states which are important to patients and which patients value. Obvious examples include being free from pain, feeling well, feeling calm, feeling that one has a good quality of life, or at least that its quality has improved and not deteriorated. Nurses come into contact with patients who are vulnerable, who suffer. An essential part of their role is to respond properly to that vulnerability and suffering.

The fact that nursing has this intrinsic ethical dimension to it is a good reason for nurses to develop their appreciation of ethical issues and also their capacity to respond properly to them. The bulk of this book is aimed towards trying to develop that capacity. But before getting on to that task it is important to say a little bit about what is involved in the capacity to appreciate the ethical dimension of practice.

If a nurse says she is unsure about how to deal with an ethical problem in her practice, it is obvious that she has already identified the problem as an *ethical* problem. So if one even gets to the stage of trying to develop responses to moral problems, one has already succeeded in identifying those problems in practice. This demonstrates that, like most of us, the nurse has the capacity of moral awareness. Without this it is not possible to recognize situations as situations with an ethical dimension to them. Such a capacity is analogous to being able to see the world in colour as opposed to seeing it in monochrome. An important realm of human life is available for us to notice – the moral realm. Awareness of the moral realm makes moral perception possible (see Blum, 1994). Moral perception occurs when we perceive of situations as having anethical dimension to them. We can also make use of the idea of moral *sensitivity*. The idea here is that some people, in contrast to others, have very good powers of moral perception. This enables such people to identify situations that have a moral dimension; only if one does this, can one respond to such situations of course.

An example might help to illustrate the point being made.

> Sandra is a nurse walking down her ward doing a 'final check' on the patients before finishing her shift. Having not noticed anything amiss, she goes in to the ward office satisfied all is well and that she can handover promptly to the nurse leading the next shift. A nursing colleague, Freda, on the same ward, is heading to the same office a second or two later. Freda notices one patient, Mrs. Jones, who is sitting up in bed, but at a slightly awkward-looking angle. Freda goes to ask Mrs. Jones if she is comfortable. She says she isn't and so Freda adjusts her pillows to make her comfortable again. Freda then proceeds to the ward office.

Let us suppose that Mrs. Jones had been in the same, slightly awkward-looking, position when Sandra walked past, but Sandra did not notice.

Freda's acts manifest sensitivity to a moral dimension of the ward area that Sandra's acts lack. This is what is meant by the kind of sensitivity being mentioned here. It is an ability to perceive moral aspects of one's environment. In the example just given, the relevant moral aspect perceived is the slight discomfort of Mrs. Jones.

A well-developed capacity of moral perception makes it much more likely that one will see relevant moral dimensions of situations in nursing practice. If one lacks this sensitivity, or one's sensitivity is insufficiently developed, one is more likely to fail to attend properly to situations of the kind under discussion here, in which a patient is in need; even if, perhaps, a relatively minor need.

It makes sense to suppose people differ in terms of the power of their moral perception. Some people's moral perception is extremely sensitive, others less so. If one thinks of moral awareness as analogous to the turning on of a light in a darkened room which makes it possible for one to see the contents of the room, those with a high degree of sensitivity see the room and its contents clearly. For those with less developed moral sensitivity the contents of the room will be less well evident. For such people the moral domain is illuminated less sharply and less extensively. Thus, Freda saw more than Sandra. Sandra did not even notice Mrs. Jones' discomfort.

In all likelihood, both nurses in the example above possessed moral awareness, and are capable of moral perception. But the moral perception of Freda is more acute – at least if we are to assess moral perception in terms of how Freda responds to Mrs. Jones' discomfort.

In addition to moral awareness, sensitivity and perception, a further component of the moral domain needs to be mentioned. This is moral imagination (Scott, 2000). What this refers to is the capacity to appreciate the significance of something as another person might see it. So, to stick with the example given above, in attempting to exercise moral imagination one might try to imagine what Mrs. Jones might be feeling. Is she thinking that she will be stuck in an uncomfortable position for several hours? From the perspective of Mrs. Jones, this is likely to have a negative effect on her overall morale. Feeling uncomfortable and being powerless to do anything about it is a terrible thing. These are the kinds of considerations which are revealed when one exercises moral imagination. The conscious exercise of moral imagination is a good way to develop one's sense of moral perception – to make it more acute, so that one is more able to identify, and thus respond to, ethical aspects of nursing practice.

So far then, we have drawn attention to the pervasiveness of ethical issues in practice, set out an argument in support of the view that nurses should study ethics, and introduced the ideas of moral awareness, sensitivity, perception and imagination. A nurse with well-developed capacities in these areas would have no difficulty in identifying ethical aspects of practice. For most of us these capacities stand in need of much further development. And also for many of us, when we first go into the clinical area it is such a strange environment that we feel our normal parameters for assessing what is right and what is wrong might not apply in this peculiar context. As mentioned above, in the clinical area one might see people who are barely clothed, who are unconscious, confused, anxious, distressed, in pain and so on. Also, whereas in ordinary life one is typically in environments that are familiar, where there are familiar expectations, none of this may be true of the clinical area. One is a novice. So all these factors can generate what might be called 'ethical disorientation'. Familiar conventions to which one is accustomed in ordinary life, such as 'wear clothes in the presence of strangers', 'don't have any physical contact with strangers', and 'don't sleep in public places' are all transgressed in the clinical area. One might suppose that since standard conventions governing behaviour don't apply in the clinical area, this is true of familiar moral strictures too. Or one may be unsure about how the ethical views one subscribes to outside the clinical area apply within it.

Here is an example to illustrate the kind of phenomenon that is being pointed to. Rhys is an inexperienced, student nurse on placement in an acute mental health admissions unit. One of the first tasks assigned to Rhys, or that he is witness to, is that of trying to rouse patients from their beds whilst they are sleep. This is the kind of task undertaken routinely, every day by the nurses who work on that unit. For them there is nothing strange about such a practice at all. But to an inexperienced nurse such as Rhys, and for most of us, this runs counter to many ethical conventions concerning, for example, privacy. Outside the clinical area it would not be appropriate for a stranger to walk into the sleeping area of another stranger, not to mention to try to wake them. Yet this is considered routine behaviour in the unit. Such events can produce the kind of ethical disorientation under discussion here. So many unusual acts are taking place – unusual by ordinary non-clinical standards – that one can become unsure of whether familiar ethical conventions apply.

If a nurse experiences this kind of thing, that is one way of identifying ethical issues in practice. Rather than to suppress the ethical rules ('dos and don'ts') which one took into the clinical area – in the above example that concerning respect for the privacy of others – one should take their transgression as an indication of the presence of an ethical issue in practice. To say that transgressing the privacy of patients and waking them from sleep is an ethical issue, is *not necessarily* to say that such acts are morally wrong. They may be perfectly justifiable, imagine there was a fire on the ward and those patients were in danger. Plainly, respecting their privacy is not as important as saving their lives. Hence experiencing moral disorientation of the kind just described is a useful indicator of an ethical issue in practice. Too often, novice nurses simply suppress their own moral intuitions assuming they must be flawed if they conflict with what is common practice in the clinical area. Rather than suppress those intuitions it is advisable to think about the nature of the conflict and try to work out which way of acting is the most ethically justified.

A further way of identifying ethical issues in practice is by using a strategy described in the next section.

How can moral issues be identified?

The kind of unease experienced by Rhys, the novice nurse we have just described, is a useful indicator of the moral dimension of practice. So as mentioned, rather than try to suppress this, it is useful to use it as a worthwhile tool to facilitate identification of moral issues in practice. In addition to this, some find the following, much more crude, strategy of help too.

Some moral issues seem easy to identify: for example, those concerning the rightness or wrongness of abortion, of mistreatment of persons with severe learning disabilities, and of injustices in the distribution of health care resources. But as we have seen moral issues pervade nursing practice. Consider the act of moving a person from one chair to another without speaking to them; removing the coat from a conscious, confused patient without their permission; preventing a confused, older patient from leaving a day care unit; trying to persuade a person with learning difficulties to have a bath, or a wash; and so on. These kinds of examples are much less likely to be cited by nursing staff as examples of moral problems encountered in practice. Yet, situations such as those just described do have a moral dimension and do raise moral questions. The following strategy is one way of trying to develop further one's sensitivity to moral issues.

The motivation for devising this strategy stemmed from speaking to student nurses who claimed never to have encountered a moral issue during their clinical placements. Undoubtedly, one has to learn to recognize such issues and in this section an attempt is made to try to outline a crude way of overcoming the difficulties which some people have in this area. The strategy has to be consciously applied and this can require a certain determination on the part of the person concerned to put the strategy into practice. Nonetheless, some nursing students (pre and post-registration) have claimed to find the strategy helpful and so it is set out below in the hope that others may find it so.

Typically, certain terms are employed, or can be employed, to describe situations with an ethical aspect. Such terms include the following:

- right
- wrong
- good
- bad
- duty
- obligation

- should

- ought

- harm

and so on. For the sake of brevity, let us refer to this list henceforth as *The List*. When one hears sentences with these terms occurring in them being used, it is likely that some kind of ethical claim is being made. For example:

- That was a good (or bad) thing to do;

- You ought to act in the best interests of your patients;

- You should have intervened when you saw a man in the street being assaulted;

- It is the duty of health care professionals to prolong life where possible;

- Nurses have an obligation to protect patients;

- Patients have a right to be told the truth about their condition;

- It is not right that some people are homeless;

and so on. These sentences each include one of the terms identified in *The List*.

Of course, some of the terms may be used in contexts which seem unrelated to ethics. For example, someone may say to a lost motorist, 'You should have turned right at the lights'. Here, the terms 'should' and 'right' occur in a context which seems not to have anything to do with ethics. However, it is plausible to hold that, in general, when the terms in the list offered above are employed, it is often the case that some kind of ethical judgement is being made. The terms in *The List* constitute indicators that an ethical claim is being made, they are not a cast-iron guarantee of the expression of such a claim. So, one way to identify situations with an ethical dimension in the health care setting is to listen out for the words in *The List*. When they are being used, or when one finds oneself using them, it is likely that some kind of ethical judgement is being made.

Clearly there are many situations which arise and about which no comments are made. For example, in a hospital ward (W ward) in the mental health context, it may be that patients are expected to queue up for their meals whilst these are served out by nursing staff. This routine may take place three times each day without anyone, nurse or patient, passing a comment upon the nature of the routine. From the fact that nobody offers a description of this routine, it does not follow that the situation lacks an ethical aspect. What this indicates is that in applying the strategy one has not simply to listen to actual descriptions of situations offered by people (colleagues, patients, patients' relatives), one must also ask the following question: Could someone describe this situation (that being witnessed, or reflected upon) in a way which involves a sentence containing one of the terms given in *The List*?

Suppose Ann is a student nurse and has been on placement at W ward for three weeks. Nobody has passed comment upon the mealtime routine just described. Suppose further that Ann decides to apply the strategy outlined above. She asks herself the question: Could someone describe this situation (patients queuing for meals which are doled out by nursing staff) in sentences which include any of the terms on *The List*? It seems plain that another person, Bethan, might say 'It's not right that patients should have to queue for their meals like that', or similarly 'It's wrong that patients are expected to queue for their meals in that way', or, again similarly, 'Patients should not be expected to queue in that way'. The possibility of Bethan legitimately making observations such as these indicates that the situation has a moral dimension. The student nurse who is applying the strategy – Ann – should then consider why Bethan's observations might be made; that is, are her comments justified?

An important point to note here is that whether or not the practice of requiring patients to queue for meals is justified, the fact that judgements such as those made by Bethan may be made about the mealtime routine on W ward indicates that the situation does have an ethical dimension. The question of whether the routine is justified from the ethical perspective is not one which we are concerned with here. Our present task is to develop and enhance the ability of nurses to identify situations with a moral dimension. In terms we used earlier, this strategy helps to enhance the moral perception of nurses. The first stage in that process involves the application of the strategy just described.

To summarize: First, one needs to listen out for the terms which feature in *The List*. If these are being employed to describe a situation (e.g., the mealtime routine on W ward), it is likely some kind of ethical claim is being made and that the situation under discussion has an ethical dimension to it. But this first step in the strategy needs to be supplemented with a second step. The person applying the strategy needs to reflect upon the situation and ask: Could someone describe this situation in sentences which include any of the terms on *The List*? Of course, it is not plausible to apply the strategy during an emergency situation, but it is possible to apply it during quieter moments in one's spell of duty, during ward-based teaching sessions, and in any period when one is reflecting upon one's work.

As noted, the conscious adoption of these strategies can enhance the development of moral perception, sensitivity, and imagination (we can assume nurses have the faculty of moral awareness). Development of moral perception can enable the nurse to appreciate more of the ethical aspects of practice. And conscious attempts at moral imagination can enhance the nurse's appreciation of the perspectives of others, both patients and colleagues. The strategies described above regarding ethical disorientation, and employment of terms in The List can help the nurse to learn to be more aware of the moral aspects of practice. The hope is that although one might have to consciously apply these strategies initially, they will gradually become part of the nurse's outlook. So that ethical aspects of practice will have due salience.

Perhaps unfortunately, learning about ethics does not provide one with ready answers to the moral problems nurses face in their daily routine. What it does do is to enable them to recognize moral problems, to have the conceptual equipment (common distinctions, knowledge of moral principles, and types of ethical theory) which can aid clear thought about them, and consequently to feel less inadequate than they otherwise would when faced with moral problems. This last point is added since many practising nurses say they feel inadequate when faced with moral problems during the course of their work. The source of this, it turns out, is often the belief that there are experts in nursing, medicine, or even moral philosophy around who know, and can prove, just what the right course of action to take in a given situation is.

Studying ethics helps to dispel this illusion and indicate to nurses that they have at least as much to offer as other groups of people in moral decision-making. In fact, the terminology of moral philosophy provides nurses with a technical vocabulary within which to couch their explanations of their own moral decisions – as might reasonably be expected of accountable professionals. It should be added that this vocabulary is one which is recognized by medical staff, health service managers, paramedics, and health economists. Hence, employing the vocabulary can help nurses to voice their concerns about relevant moral matters in an effective way.

There is a useful passage from Seedhouse (1988, p. 64) which we might briefly consider:

> The realistic aim of ethical inquiry is to clarify the issues, to show those who have to make decisions the full range of possibilities open to them, and to explain different perspectives and ways of reasoning.

Seedhouse indicates here that ethics, when applied to the health care context, has very modest aims; it cannot provide uniquely and indisputably correct solutions to moral problems. This is simply not feasible.

The chapter can be drawn to a close by making a quite general point. It was noted earlier that actions which result in harms or benefits to others form a major part of the subject matter of ethics. Since the point of health care is to promote the well-being of patients – to undertake actions which result in benefits to others – it is plausible to hold that every nursing action has an ethical dimension. This point underlies Seedhouse's slogan 'Work for health is a moral endeavour' (1988, p. 17). Since, presumably, all nursing actions – filling in records, interacting with patients and so on – are ultimately undertaken for their benefit, it is evident that Seedhouse's slogan is appropriate. It is true that some actions undertaken by nurses may involve causing harm to patients. Perhaps giving people medication against their will is an example, as is giving medication by injection. But these harm-causing actions are only justifiably undertaken if in doing so more benefits, or fewer harms, result.

Conclusion

This introductory chapter has drawn attention to the inherent ethical dimension of nursing practice, described the concepts of moral awareness, perception, sensitivity, and imagination, and offered a strategy for both the identification of ethical issues in practice and also the development of moral sensitivity, perception and imagination. Having done all this, it is necessary in the next chapter to begin to introduce the approach to be put forward here for addressing ethical issues in practice.

Chapter 2

Judgements, Rules, Principles and Theories

In the previous chapter, we looked briefly at the nature of ethics and a strategy was offered for the identification of moral issues which occur in nursing practice. We also highlighted the importance of moral awareness, perception and imagination. In the present chapter and the next, a framework for moral reasoning is set out. This chapter outlines the main elements of that framework. As we will see, it comprises of four 'levels', each of which concerns either judgements, rules, principles or theories. The four moral principles of respect for autonomy, beneficence, non-maleficence and justice are introduced in this chapter and then described fully in the next. The relationship between the various levels of the framework is also explained. In the final section of the chapter it will be argued that level three of the framework (that concerning the four principles) captures the most important level of moral thinking for our purposes. This prepares the ground for a fuller exposition of the principles in Chapter 3.

Moral judgements

A rough distinction can be drawn between four levels of thinking about moral matters. The first level consists of moral judgements, the second of moral rules, the third of moral principles, and the fourth of moral theories (Beauchamp and Childress, 1989, p. 6). We can begin to explain these by looking at 'level-one' moral judgements.

These are judgements about a particular situation; they are made by those involved in the situation, those who witness the situation or those who simply read or come to hear about it. One example of a moral judgement would be a decision by a nurse to withhold information from a patient. Perhaps the patient asks the nurse for information concerning the side effects of medication presently being prescribed. The nurse might judge that the right thing to do here is to withhold this information on the grounds that if the patient learns the truth he might refuse to take the medication with the probable consequence that the patient's health will worsen.

Another example of a particular moral judgement is a nurse's judgement that the patient's request for information concerning the side effects of the medication should be responded to in a different way. The considerations of the previous chapter support the conclusion that all actions undertaken by nursing staff have a moral dimension. This shows that all decisions or judgements made by nurses also have a moral dimension since they always affect, directly or indirectly, the health of patients. In the example just given, the nurse is required to make a particular moral judgement: should the patient be given the information requested or not? A situation such as this demands that the nurse makes a moral judgement.

It might be suggested that the nurse could simply avoid making a judgement, perhaps by informing the patient that he or she (the nurse) does not have the information, or is not able to give the information. But even strategies such as these have a moral dimension to them since, presumably, the nurse thinks that either the patient or the nurse will be harmed if the information is given (perhaps the nurse has been 'instructed' by senior colleagues not to give the information to the patient). The point is that even a judgement not to make a decision – an evasion, so to speak – is also a decision to act in a way which has a moral dimension. This is due to the fact that considerations involving possible harms and benefits, either to the patient or the nurse concerned, enter into the rationale for the decision and result from it.

The example just discussed illustrates what is meant by a moral judgement. Consider, now, moral rules.

Moral rules

Moral rules are to be found in the kinds of instructions which are familiar to all of us. Parents typically try to instil such rules in their children, so they will behave well, and develop into good people. They include such rules as 'don't lie', 'don't hurt others', 'don't steal', 'be truthful', 'try to be good', 'do your best', 'keep promises', 'don't cheat' and so on. It is clear that these rules are not absolute, they can be broken if there is good reason to do so. If telling someone the truth will cause them a great deal of pain, then two moral rules come into conflict: 'be truthful', and 'don't hurt others'. In such conflicts we might decide that one rule is more important than another, and so we might decide that, on this occasion, it is more important not to hurt the other person than it is to be truthful with them. Such a decision illustrates the way in which rules can conflict, and also the way in which rules can be broken if there are sufficient moral grounds to do so. Beauchamp and Childress (2009, p. 15) employ the term *prima facie* (literally: 'at first sight') to capture this feature of rules – their 'breachability' as we might put it. 'At first sight' one should respect moral rules, unless, given further thought, other considerations stemming from other moral rules are more pressing.

Here are two further points. The first is that a particular moral judgement is an instance of a moral rule. The relationship between rules and their instances can be explained as follows. Suppose one is driving a car and stops at a red light. This particular act of stopping at a red light is an instance of the driver obeying the rule 'Stop at red lights'. So, for example, by not lying to a person, or telling the truth to them, one is instantiating the general rules 'It is wrong to lie', or, 'One ought to be truthful'.

The second point is that level-two rules provide justification for level-one judgements. Hence, if asked to justify an act of telling a patient the truth (as in our earlier example), a nurse may say that one ought to tell the truth, or it is wrong to lie to others. The nurse appeals to level-two rules as justifications for the act – the act of telling the truth.

The moral rules given above illustrate the difference between rules and judgements. They are basic moral rules that are passed on to children in many cultures. They are part of what might be called 'the common morality' (Beauchamp and Childress, 2009, p. 3). But our concerns are, of course, narrower than the common morality since our focus is on ethics in nursing practice. So when considering which, if any, moral rules are most relevant to nursing practice, the rules will be selected with the particular parameters of nursing practice in mind.

In their discussion, Beauchamp and Childress highlight four moral rules which they hold to be of particular significance to the ethical dimension of the relationship between health care professionals and patients. The four they highlight are rules of veracity, privacy, confidentiality and fidelity (2009, p. 288). Before proceeding to discuss each of these, it is worth just pausing to consider why these four, in particular, are highlighted in their discussion. The rationale seems to be that the obligations captured by these four rules can be subsumed under one or more of the four principles (of which more below). So that explains why the four rules are presented as rules as opposed to principles. But still an explanation is lacking as to why these particular four are selected, one might have added a 'consent rule' for example (see Beauchamp and Childress, 2009, p. 13). What is clear, though, is that the content of any important moral obligations which happen to fall outside these four rules will have to be covered by one or more of the moral principles or theories we discuss later. Otherwise, the approach will be seriously incomplete. Having made this point, we now proceed to describe the four rules which Beauchamp and Childress single out for special attention; as mentioned; these are the veracity rule, the privacy rule, the confidentiality rule and the fidelity rule.

Veracity rule

The veracity rule concerns obligations on the part of nurses to be truthful in their dealings with patients. Part of this involves giving information and doing so in such a way that patients can understand it. As will be seen later, the moral significance of veracity stems from its relationship to the moral principle of respect for autonomy and so more light will be cast on the rule later when we discuss that principle. But for now it can be pointed out that truth-telling in the nurse–patient relationship is an important aspect of it. Patients often rely on nurses to give them information about their care, their diagnosis, prognosis, medication and so on. This is the case even though medical staff do these things too. Patients may be given information by a doctor and then after having thought about it, the patient may raise questions about the information with a nurse. This is a very important part of nurse–patient interactions, as patients often rely on nurses to facilitate their own understanding of facts relevant to their care. Also, it is common to point out that trust is an important aspect of the nurse–patient relationship, and truth-telling seems bound up with that (de Raeve, 2002). To describe a relationship as trusting is to imply that each partner is truthful with the other. Imagine some one saying 'I trust my partner, though he tells me many lies and I am never sure whether what he says to me is true'. Is that coherent? Surely such a relationship is characterized by suspicion, not trust. Certainly it seems plausible to think that trust and truthfulness go together.

Privacy rule

Beauchamp and Childress define privacy as 'a state or condition of limited access [to a person]' (2009, p. 296). So a moral rule embodying the value of privacy would express an obligation to respect privacy. We can point to at least four ways in which such obligations can be interpreted.

The first is the most obvious, that is simply the obligation to respect the personal space of others. Hence, a moral rule to respect the privacy of others refers to the obligation to respect their 'personal space'. This can be understood quite literally, in terms of an obligation not to encroach upon a person – perhaps by entering the person's home without invitation. This kind of application of the privacy rule can be illustrated in the context of caring for people with learning disabilities. For example, as some new community home is opened – perhaps one which contains some special facility – processions of visitors might be shown around the new home. Such visitors may include local dignitaries or other workers in the field of learning disabilities. It is plausible that such visits constitute violations of the privacy rule in this first sense. (Think how most people would respond to having strangers shown around their homes.) And of course, in the context of ward-based nursing, one respects the privacy of patients by drawing curtains around their bed when they are being treated, for example.

Second, respecting the privacy of the person can take the form of restricting access to information about the person. So, for example, a nurse who gives out information concerning a patient without their permission can plausibly be regarded as breaching the privacy of that patient. This second aspect of the privacy rule is, of course, closely related and probably overlaps with the confidentiality rule (see below).

A third understanding of privacy is that in the sense of 'decisional privacy' (Beauchamp and Childress, 2009, p. 296). This evidently points to obligations to respect rights to make decisions without intrusion. So a nurse who intrudes upon a discussion between a patient and their spouse about treatment options, for example, would transgress their privacy in this sense.

A final understanding of privacy is that of 'proprietary privacy' (Beauchamp and Childress, 2009, p. 296). This concerns, for example, claims to ownership of one's tissues, such as genetic material, or blood samples. It may be considered important that tissue donors retain some degree of control over what is done to their human tissue even though it has been removed from their body with their permission (see Human Tissue Act, 2004).

What needs to be stressed again is that, as with all the rules being discussed here (and the principles to be discussed shortly), the obligations captured in them are *prima facie* and not absolute, as explained earlier. Thus suppose a nurse suspects that a patient is having a cardiac arrest but is hidden from view by screens because the patient had earlier requested some privacy. In such circumstances the obligation to save the life of the patient by administration of cardio-pulmonary respiration (CPR) is more important than the obligation to respect the patient's privacy. (Of course the example assumes there to be no unusual aspects to this case: the patient's prognosis is good and he has not made any prior requests about non-treatment.)

Confidentiality rule

The idea of what would count as a failure to respect confidentiality is described in the following: 'An infringement of a person's right to confidentiality occurs only if the person (or institution) to whom the information was disclosed in confidence fails to protect the information or deliberately discloses it to someone without first-party consent' (Beauchamp and Childress, 2009, pp. 302–3).

Thus we have two ways in which breaches of confidentiality are identified in this definition. The first occurs when there is a failure to protect the information given in confidence. The second occurs where confidential information is actually disclosed without the consent of the patient.

So, suppose a patient tells Sandra, a nurse, in confidence that she was sexually abused as a child. With the agreement of the patient, Sandra records this information in her case notes. It is plain that others in the health care team have access to the information since they have legitimate access to the patient's case notes too. Again, suppose the patient is made aware of this. So far no breach of confidentiality occurs. Suppose, now, though that Sandra discusses the patient's history with a friend, including the details about her sexual abuse. Now confidentiality in the second of the senses we identified is breached. This is because Sandra disclosed the information about the patient to someone who has no connection with the care of the patient, and did so without the consent of the patient.

To illustrate how breaches of confidentiality in the first sense described might arise, suppose also that during the course of her shift during the day, Sandra had left the notes she made from her discussions with the patient about the abuse on a chair by the patient's bed. One of the patient's visitors then comes across them and reads them. She is shocked to learn about what has happened to her friend in the past. By failing to protect the information properly, Sandra breaches confidentiality in this way too. (The patient's privacy is also violated here.)

To illustrate how a distinction can be drawn between breaches of privacy on one hand, and of confidentiality on the other, suppose the information about the patient is now placed on the hospital trust's patient database. A computer hacker breaks into the database. Upon noticing a name familiar to her, she too reads information about our patient's history of abuse. The hacker is failing to respect the privacy of the patient, and also of the privacy of any of the other patients whose records she reads. Neither the hospital trust nor the health care professionals themselves are guilty of breaching the confidentiality of the patient in such a case. This is so, provided they safeguarded the information properly and did not disclose it to parties unconnected to the care of the patient.

Fidelity rule

The fidelity rule concerns obligations 'to act in good faith, to keep vows and promises, fulfil agreements, maintain relationships and discharge fiduciary relationships' (Beauchamp and Childress, 2001, p. 312, 2009, p. 311). One gets something of the sense of the obligations that this rule intends to capture by recalling that the term 'fidelity' derives from the Latin term '*fide*' meaning 'faithful' (hence 'Fido' was once a popular name for dogs). In the context of nursing care this is a reminder that the relationship between nurses and patients has a special character to it. It is not on a par with the relationship between a customer (the patient) and a supplier (the nurse). Due to the inherent vulnerability of the patient, a commitment on the part of a nurse to do her best for the patient ought to be an intrinsic part of the nurse–patient relationship. The obligations of fidelity are intended to capture these.

An example might help. Rupa is a nurse working in the community. Early in her working day, she receives a call from an elderly patient, who sounds as though he is in some distress. The patient assures Rupa that he is not in immediate danger but would like to see Rupa sometime that day. Rupa assures the patient that although she has other patients to see, she will definitely find time to visit the patient to get a fuller picture of what is going on with him. However, Rupa's day turns out to be unexpectedly hectic, she has to find a place in sheltered accommodation for one of her patients and other patients occupy a lot of her time, much more than she had anticipated. Before she realizes, it is 7.00 p.m. and she is exhausted. Not only that, she has completely forgotten about her pledge to visit the patient who phoned her at the start of the day.

The obligations captured in the fidelity rule are involved in this example. To start with, there is an *implicit* commitment from the nurse to the patient stemming from the fact that he is one of Rupa's patients. Moreover, she makes an *explicit* commitment to go to see the patient that day, which as we saw, she fails to fulfil. This would be a failure to observe the fidelity rule, at least in terms of the obligations to the patient discussed above. Of course, Rupa has fulfilled many other obligations to her other patients. But the patient who she did not get around to seeing – having pledged to do so – is likely to feel let down by Rupa. To say all this, is not necessarily to imply that Rupa has behaved unethically. Recall again the point about the obligations which are captured in rules having only 'prima facie' binding. It may be that her other patients were in much greater need than the patient she spoke to on the phone. If so, it may be that her decision to give more time to them, at the expense of the other patient is morally justified, even if she *had* remembered giving the assurance to the patient that she would go to see him. The main purpose of the example is to highlight the kinds of moral obligations captured in the fidelity rule.

Another example of situations in which there are implicit commitments on the part of nurses to patients arises in contexts in which patients give information about themselves to nurses. They give information such as their age, next of kin and so forth, on the tacit understanding that the nurse concerned will convey the information only to parties who have a legitimate interest – namely, other health care professionals (medical staff, other nurses and so on).

Further, it is plausible to note that patients assume that nursing staff are committed to undertake their duties with the required degree of skill and care, to provide them with relevant information and not to be wilfully negligent. These things are simply presupposed by patients in their dealings with nurses. Also, the fidelity rule covers a very general obligation to respect the relevant professional standards, for example those set out in the NMC Code (2008; see Appendix).

These, then, are the four level-two moral rules identified by Beauchamp and Childress. It should be clear that the example of a moral rule such as 'It is wrong to lie' can be subsumed within the veracity rule; so too can rules such as, 'One ought, in general, to tell the truth'. We will return in Chapter 3 to comment on the relationship between level-two moral rules and clauses in the NMC Code (NMC, 2008). Before this, it is necessary to look, briefly, at four level-three principles (these are to be set out more fully in Chapter 3), and then at three moral theories.

Moral principles

In Beauchamp and Childress's approach, four moral principles play a central role. These are the principle of respect for *autonomy,* the principle of *beneficence,* the principle of *non-maleficence,* and the principle of *justice.* Principles are said to be more general than moral rules. For example, the principle of non-maleficence refers to obligations not to cause harm. This is clearly more general than specific moral rules such as do not burn others; do not hit them, do not kick them, and so on. So the sense in which principles are more general than rules seems fairly easy to grasp.

Summarily stated, the principle of respect for *autonomy* refers to obligations to respect the choices which others make concerning their own lives. Hence, if a patient chooses, on the basis of relevant information, not to take medication prescribed, then obligations referred to by the principle of respect for autonomy point to an obligation on the part of others to respect that choice. Obligations regarding information giving also form part of what is required by this principle.

The principle of *beneficence* refers to obligations to act in ways which promote the well-being of others. It is clear that construed in this way, this principle is of central relevance to the nursing context and, more generally, to all health care workers. As we saw in Chapter 1, one important goal of nursing actions is to promote the well-being of patients and, hence, to act beneficiently.

The principle of *non-maleficence* refers to obligations not to harm others. This differs from beneficence in the sense that it imposes fewer obligations on us. For example, suppose again that one is walking down a city street and one sees a person who is obviously thin, unhealthy and hungry. The principle of beneficence obliges one to help this person, to act in ways which will benefit him. But non-maleficence is less morally demanding, so to speak: it only concerns obligations not to harm the person. The distinction between the principles of beneficence and non-maleficence has quite serious implications for health care professionals. A fundamental aim of health care is, as suggested above, to promote the well-being of people. Hence, as we noted, the actions of nursing staff can be said to be grounded in beneficence. So it is reasonable to conclude that regimes of care should actually benefit patients, rather than simply not cause harm to them. Thus, regimes of care which merely prevent harm coming to their patients fall short of what is required by the principle of beneficence.

The fourth and final level-four principle to be defined briefly here is the principle of *justice*. This principle refers to obligations to treat others fairly. On one construal, this principle asserts that equals be treated equally and unequals unequally (Beauchamp and Childress, 2009, p. 242). So, in the nursing context, suppose in one set of circumstances a nurse tells the truth to a patient, Colin, at his request, concerning the nature of his condition. Later, another patient, Charles, whose circumstances are the same as Colin's makes a similar request. This time the nurse is not truthful with the patient and does not give Charles the information he requests (it is to be assumed that the nurse has time to speak to Charles). Since the situations of Colin and Charles in our example are the same, Charles may claim that he has not been treated fairly and that the principle of justice has been transgressed in the sense that equals have not been responded to equally.

Also, the concept of justice arises fundamentally in decisions involving resource allocation. For obvious reasons questions of justice in that context are said to involve the concept of *distributive* justice, since they involve questions about the distribution of a good, the 'good' referred to here is that of health care itself.

Before closing this introductory summary of the four principles, it is necessary to consider a proposal that a fifth principle should be added to the four which feature so prominently in Beauchamp and Childress's approach. The fifth principle would be a principle of respect for *persons*. The rationale for expanding the four in this way stems from the recognition that if it is accepted that all human beings are persons, not all persons are autonomous. Thus babies, people with senile dementia, those with very severe mental health problems, and people with very severe intellectual disabilities, it may be said, lack the capacity to be autonomous. Hence, it may be pointed out, the principle of respect for autonomy does not apply to them, and so they are at risk of moral neglect in some way.

However, the list of principles will not be expanded here to include that of respect for persons, for three main reasons. First, if asked to explain just what is involved in such respect, one is led to try to make sense of the idea by appealing to expressions such as 'to have moral regard for'. So, the view would be, even if one cannot respect the autonomy of non-autonomous persons, one should have moral regard for them. In the context of health care, I take it to be too obvious to be worth stating that one should have moral regard for those one comes into contact with – be they patients, their relatives, colleagues or any other human being. If one does not have moral regard for others, one should not be a nurse (or any other kind of health care professional). So this is one reason for avoiding the addition of this fifth principle. The second reason is this. When one tries to tease out further just what it is to 'have moral regard' for persons, I think one is led to explain this in terms of moral concepts that are captured in the principles. Thus to have regard for them is make sure they don't come to harm, that their best interests are protected, and that they are treated fairly. The third reason is one offered by Beauchamp and Childress themselves (2009, p. 70). This is that over the past 30 years or so a distinction has been drawn between persons and human beings (see Harris, 1985). Roughly, the proposal is that only beings who are able to reason count as persons. Thus, babies, those with severe dementia, patients in persistent vegetative states, are human beings but not persons. This has prompted discussion and debate about the very nature of what it is to be a person and indeed whether it is plausible to distinguish between human beings who are persons, on the one hand, and human beings who are not persons on the other. In the context of a discussion of nursing ethics I take this to be beyond our current concerns in this book. Whether a patient counts as a person or not they need to be given due care, and such care must meet the requirements set in the standards of conduct for members of the nursing profession. So for these three reasons we will not expand the list of principles to five. Even though the principle of respect for autonomy might not apply to patients who are not autonomous, the obligations referred to by the other principles still do so there should be no risk of neglect of such patients, to do so would be to fail to respect one's obligations of non-maleficence, beneficence or justice to such patients.

This brings to a close our preliminary introduction to the four level-three moral principles. Moving on, three level-four moral theories will now be discussed, specifically: (a) Utilitarianism, (b) a Kantian duty-based or deontological theory, and (c) virtue theory.

Moral theories: utilitarianism, deontology, virtue theory

Utilitarianism

We can identify three influential moral theories: first, a theory which focuses upon the consequences of actions and which, hence, can be described as consequence-based; second, a theory which focuses on moral duty and which can be described as duty-based; and a third one which focuses on virtue and can be described as virtue-based. The first of these theories is termed Utilitarianism (two of its most famous proponents were J. Bentham [1748–1832] and J. S. Mill [1808–73]).

A nurse who is a Utilitarian would base a decision concerning which course of action to take in response to a moral problem entirely on consideration of the consequences of those actions. According to the Utilitarian approach to ethics, in the event of there being a choice between two or more possible courses of action, the morally right act is that which results in the greatest 'good'. By 'good', here, is meant, for example pleasure, or happiness. So, if one act, A, will result in more pleasure than another act, B, then one ought to do A.

In cases where all conceivable courses of action are likely to result in some degree of pain (say, the case of a terminally ill person who is in constant pain; or a person with mental health problems who is tormented by hallucinations), Utilitarianism demands that the morally right act is that which results in the least amount of harms, hence the least amount of pain.

So, according to Utilitarians, acts are morally right to the extent that they either maximize a good (say, happiness) or minimize a harm (say, pain). This is captured in the so-called principle of utility:

> [Actions] are right in proportion as they tend to promote happiness, wrong as they tend to produce the reverse of happiness. By happiness is intended pleasure, and the absence of pain; by unhappiness, pain and the privation of pleasure. (Mill, 1863, p. 257)

Consider three points in favour of Utilitarianism. First, the approach seeks to establish a quantifiable basis for moral decision-making by employing a kind of calculation. Hence, moral decision-making would not be a matter of arbitrary opinion, but would be based on calculation. Thus, suppose it could be shown that compulsory treatment for anorexic patients leads to greater levels of overall happiness than is produced by other means. From a Utilitarian perspective, compulsory treatment is the more morally justified therapeutic response.

Second, the claim that acts are morally right if they maximize happiness or minimize suffering seems, at least at first sight, to be a plausible one. Most of us would agree that happiness is a good thing which should be increased, and that suffering is bad and should be reduced.

Third, a further consideration in support of Utilitarianism is this. As we will see shortly, in duty-based ethical theory, one of the most important duties is the duty not to lie. However, there seem to be occasions where one might well think it is justified to tell a lie. Thus consider a situation in which a person, A, intends to injure another person, B; you know where B is; you also know that if you reveal B's whereabouts, then B will take a severe beating. It seems justified in such a case to lie to A, to protect B – especially if you know that in an hour or so A will have calmed down and will not want to assault B. An apparent advantage of Utilitarianism is that some flexibility appears to be present in such cases. If it is the case that lying results in more overall happiness, then we would be justified in lying. So, in our example, it would be acceptable to lie and so save B from a beating.

These three sets of considerations indicate that Utilitarianism has at least initial plausibility. It is common to distinguish two forms of Utilitarianism: Act Utilitarianism and Rule Utilitarianism.

Act Utilitarianism

Act Utilitarians consider only the consequences of one act at a time. So, when they face a moral dilemma, they will simply calculate which of the possible acts will maximize benefits or minimize harms. So, suppose a nurse who is desperate for money to repay some debts steals money from a confused patient. Suppose further that neither the patient nor any other person ever realizes what has happened to the money. If the nurse is confident that the patient would not miss the money, would not suffer as a result of its being taken, and that no one else would notice either, it seems to follow that stealing the money is justifiable from a Utilitarian perspective. This is because the act of stealing the money leads to greater overall levels of happiness. In particular, the nurse experiences greater level of happiness than if she had not stolen the money and no other person is any worse off.

One might think, though, that the fact that the performance of such an apparently unethical act as that just described seems justifiable in Act Utilitarianism appears to constitute a powerful criticism of it; it is surely morally abhorrent to steal from a vulnerable, confused patient even if nobody else ever discovers the crime and the patient himself never becomes aware of it.

However, another form of Utilitarianism – Rule Utilitarianism – has been proposed to overcome the kind of objection presented by the 'unscrupulous nurse' case.

Rule Utilitarianism

In response to the unscrupulous nurse example it may be pointed out that although stealing from the patient maximized utility on that one occasion, if it became known that nurses would exploit patients in such an objectionable manner then this would lead to very many undesirable consequences – lots of unhappiness. So, since preserving trust in the nurse–patient relationship is a good thing, it maximizes happiness, then a moral rule such as 'never steal from patients' maximizes overall utility even though in some instances it might cause unhappiness to some desperate impoverished nurses. Thus the Rule Utilitarin seeks to identify and propose general rules adherence to which maximizes overall utility.

Similarly, although Act Utilitarianism justifies lying on a specific occasion if this produces more happiness than truth-telling if it became known that nurses could not be trusted to be truthful to patients, trust in the nurse–patient relationship might be eroded. Thus, the Rule Utilitarian may propose that nurses should be truthful in their dealings with their patients. The reason, it may be said, is that patients are more likely to trust health care professionals if they are sure that they are honest and truthful. In this case, they will be more likely to impart relevant information and hold such professionals in high regard. It can be supposed that these consequences of being truthful are beneficial (they maximize happiness), since health care professionals often require information in order to treat patients successfully; and if they are held in high regard, their views are likely to be respected. So, even if on a particular occasion being truthful with a patient leads to more harmful than beneficial consequences, the net benefits of being truthful in most cases would be claimed to outweigh the net harms.

It is therefore conceivable that a Rule Utilitarian may tell the truth to a patient even if, on that occasion, doing so leads to more harms than benefits. They would do so on the grounds that adherence to a moral rule, which requires that one is truthful with others, generally leads to more benefits than harms. However, critics point out that it is difficult to see how Rule Utilitarinism can qualify as a version of Utilitarianism if it allows one to act in ways which will not maximize utility.

Having looked at the general character of Utilitarianism, and also at the distinction between Act and Rule Utilitarianism, some of the common criticisms of this theory will now be considered.

Criticism of Utilitarianism

Although Utilitarianism claims to provide a secure, calculable basis for moral decision-making, it is hard to see how this can be achieved. It is of course notoriously difficult to determine the consequences of particular acts or of the adoption of general rules. For example, suppose an Act Utilitarian refrains from telling the truth to a patient on the grounds that to do so would lead to overall disutility. Suppose, for example, that one of the patient's children has died unknown to the patient, and the Utilitarian nurse, believing that the patient has only a few days to live, does not want to burden the patient with this news even when he is asked by him if his children are well. If the patient were to get better, he might become extremely distressed about the fact that he was lied to; and this may sour the future relationship between health care professionals and that patient.

Second, Williams (1972) argues that Utilitarianism is morally debasing. Since its sole aim is the maximizing of pleasure (or minimizing of pain), in principle, any kind of act could be said to be morally right. The point being, here, that in some other moral theories certain types of acts are claimed to be absolutely wrong, with a clear restriction on what is permissible. In Utilitarianism, however, the overriding consideration is maximizing utility, so that it is possible that an act which might be considered morally abhorrent would be morally permissible in Utilitarianism – even torturing babies or young children. Nothing is ruled out.

Third, Williams points out that from the Utilitarian perspective certain acts seem obviously right even though for most of us they would seem highly controversial and not clear cut at all. For example, suppose one could save the lives of ten people but only by killing one person. Even if that is indeed morally right, Williams wonders whether it is *obviously* right (Williams, cited in Smart and Williams, 1973, p. 98).

Fourth, of course, it is highly problematic to quantify phenomena such as pleasure or pain. It looks very difficult, perhaps impossible, to assess that action x produces, say, 20 units of happiness, in contrast to action y which produces only 13, and that therefore action x is the right one to perform.

Also, recall our unscrupulous nurse example, for most of us it seems simply outrageous to steal from a vulnerable patient in the way described above. We think this irrespective of the consequences of acting in such a way. Whether or not the patient, or anyone else, would come to realize that their money had been stolen, we would want to say the nurse acted wrongly. But in an approach which defines the rightness and wrongness of acts solely in terms of their consequences, Utilitarianism, in both Act and Rule versions, lacks the moral resources to register this problem with it.

Lastly, as can be shown by a more extreme version of our 'unscrupulous nurse' example, critics of Utilitarianism complain that it can justify morally abhorrent practices such as slavery. If the misery of the slaves is outweighed by the happiness of the slave owners then slavery looks morally justified from a Utilitarian perspective. If anything is wrong, surely slavery is wrong.

So, in spite of initial attractions, it appears that there are serious problems with Utilitarianism. The theory we consider next captures the intuition, raised by the unscrupulous nurse example, that some actions are so unethical it can never be morally right to perform them.

Deontological theory

Deontological moral theories take duty to be the basis of morality. Perhaps the most well-known form of deontological moral theory is that proposed by Immanuel Kant (1724–1804). His view is stated in his *Groundwork of the Metaphysic of Morals*, which can be found in Paton's translation (Kant, 1948). (For references to other versions of deontological theories see Singer, 1991.) Kant is without doubt one of the most important of philosophers but his work is notoriously difficult and there are various interpretations of it.

From our point of view, Kant's theory has relevance due to its emphasis on moral duty where this is considered apart from consequences. As noted, many of us think that certain kinds of actions are definitely morally wrong, regardless of their consequences. We considered just such an example in our discussion of the unscrupulous nurse. Another example might be the sexual abuse of young children. For many, there can be no justification for such acts. It seems to be a severe weakness of Utilitarianism that no type of action is definitely ruled out; as we saw, this is because in Utilitarianism the overriding consideration concerns the maximization of utility.

Kant's moral theory begins from an acceptance of the view that there is a moral theory currently in place; that is, there is a moral system which people generally employ – call this the 'commonsense' theory, or 'ordinary moral thought'. His view seems to be that any moral theory should begin from consideration of the main components of the commonsense theory. So, for Kant, there is an existing moral system in place which people apply, in rough and ready fashion, in their ordinary dealings with each other. What he seeks to do is to propose a moral theory which rests upon fundamental components of this ongoing, commonsense theory. As Kant puts it:

> The sole aim of the present Groundwork is to seek out and establish *the supreme principle of morality*...The method I have adopted...[proceeds] analytically from common knowledge to the foundation of its supreme principle and then back again synthetically from an examination of this principle and its origins to the common knowledge in which we find its application. (Kant, 1948, pp. 57–8; also Raphael, 1981, p. 58)

Kant notes that there is a distinction present in ordinary moral thought, and regarded as important within such thought, between acts which are done out of respect for duty on the one hand, and acts done either from what he calls inclination or acts done from prudential considerations (acting out of self-interest) on the other. Kant's view can be put thus:

> A human action is morally good, not because it is done from immediate inclination – still less because it is done from self-interest – but because it is done for the sake of duty. (Kant, 1948, p. 19, summarizing Kant's view)

So, in the following three cases, there is an important moral difference between the actors:

1. A person, A, who whilst acting out of respect for duty, performs an act of type X because he takes it to be the case that he has a duty to do X – regardless of the consequences (as in the case of truth-telling, for example). Thus suppose that A is a student nurse Alan, who notices that a severely physically disabled patient has been incontinent and acts to make the patient comfortable by helping him to change into dry clothing. Alan does this act out of recognition of a moral duty to help people unable to help themselves where possible.

2. A person, B, who performs an act of type X (as before, telling the truth, or being honest) merely out of convenience and not out of any particular recognition of a duty to do X (to be truthful). Such a person is said by Kant to be acting out of inclination (1948, p. 63). He may do X just as person, A, above, but although his action conforms with duty, it is not done out of respect for duty. For example, suppose that Alan had made the patient referred to in case (1) comfortable simply to fill in some time and not from of an intention to act morally: Alan's action would conform with moral duty, but would not be undertaken out of respect for moral duty.

3. A person, C, who performs an act of type X for purely prudential reasons – purely from self-interest. Kant gives the example of a shopkeeper who is honest because he or she fears that there may be adverse consequences of not being honest – the acquiring of a bad reputation and loss of business, for example (1948, p. 63). Such a person is honest only because of calculating the consequences of not being honest, and concluding that it is not in their best interests to be dishonest. Again, of such a person, it can be claimed that what they do conforms with duty but is not done out of respect for duty. Another example would be a student nurse who makes comfortable the patient referred to in cases (1) and (2) simply to impress the senior nurse; this would qualify as acting out of self-interest rather than from moral duty.

Kant suggests, plausibly, that an important moral difference can be identified between the actor in (1) on the one hand, and the actors in (2) and (3) on the other. What is central to the distinction are the intentions of the actors: A intends to act out of respect for moral duty but this is not the case with B and C. Kant especially seeks to emphasize the difference between A and C. C's decision to act honestly is the consequence of reasoning *hypothetically*. That is, he reasons thus: 'if I do X the consequences will be Y; if I do not do X, the consequences will be Z. Since I desire Y, I'll do X'. In the case of A, however, Kant points out that he does not go through such a reasoning process; A simply reasons thus: 'it is my duty to do X, therefore I ought to do X'.

A central component in Kant's theory is the concept of *autonomy* (1948, p. 93), and it is important to say a few words about this before continuing. As noted, Kant takes as fundamental the distinction between acting out of respect for duty, and merely acting in conformity with it. To be capable of acting out of respect for duty it is necessary that the person is free to decide to act in such a way. So, Kant's view requires that what he calls 'the will' (the mind) is actually free to make moral decisions, or to put the same point another way, to be capable of acting morally or immorally it is necessary that one is capable of deciding to undertake acts in the first place. Only 'autonomous' beings are thus capable.

This should be easy for us to accept: ordinary moral thought distinguishes an act done voluntarily, from one done as a result of coercion. For example, suppose two people donate half of their savings to a worthwhile charity. It is later discovered that one did this of her own free will whilst the other did it because he was under some kind of threat – suppose he was blackmailed into donating the sum to charity. Commonsense moral thinking would distinguish between the two acts: the view being that the voluntary donation is the more worthy act from the moral perspective. This example indicates the central position which the notion of autonomy has in moral thinking.

A further point which needs to be mentioned here is that in drawing the distinction between hypothetical and categorical reasoning, the person who reasons hypothetically takes into consideration facts which for Kant are not relevant to the question of the rightness or otherwise of the particular act. Instead of simply thinking about what is his duty to do, the subject who reasons hypothetically considers the consequences of his act. For Kant, thinking in such a way constitutes a threat to the person's autonomy; when subjects 'look beyond' the question of what is right or wrong and begin to consider the consequences of their acts they are not thinking morally – he says they are looking for 'inducements' (1948, p. 67) to act morally; and moral actions are not undertaken out of consideration of 'inducements'. Hence, the difference between Kant's duty-based approach to ethics, and the Utilitarian approach can be seen to be extremely profound.

The categorical imperative

Kant takes it to be the case that acting morally is essentially bound up with acting out of respect for duty. In fact, he is claiming that it is a necessary condition of moral actions that they are carried out due to recognition of duty. Given this claim, then, concerning the necessity of the notion of duty to moral acts, the question arises of which particular duties we ought to decide, as individual autonomous persons, to respect. (Bear in mind that for Kant these have to be worked out for oneself.)

Kant claims that we can determine what our duty is by applying the categorical imperative. It is 'categorical' because it admits of no exceptions; and it is 'imperative' because it is necessary – according to Kant – to act out of respect for it. One formulation of this is as follows:

> I ought never to act except in such a way that I can also will that my maxim should become a universal law. (Kant, 1948, p. 67)

Less formally: do unto others as you would have them do unto you. So, crudely, the claim is that one should only perform an act of type X (telling a lie; breaking a promise) if one is prepared to allow that every other person in similar circumstances should necessarily perform the same type of act.

In illustration of this idea Kant discusses the case of a person who is considering making a promise that she knows she is not able to keep (1948, p. 67). Suppose they try to work out what moral duty demands of them. To do this, they ask if the rule ('maxim' in Kant's words) 'it is right to escape a difficulty by making a false promise' can be a coherent universal law. It will be one which applies to all other people – will be *universalized* in Kant's terms. Kant thinks such a rule could not be universalized into a coherent universal law. This is because if everyone made such false promises, the promises would obviously not be believed, because everyone would know them to be false promises, not genuine ones. So if you were to lend money to the person who promises to repay it you would be very silly since you will be doing so in the knowledge that the person has no intention of repaying it. Hence the very practice of 'promising' in this context would be devoid of meaning. This is what Kant is getting at in suggesting that it is not even coherent to universalize the rule: 'escape a difficulty by making a false promise'. To universalize it would be to end the practice of promising.

He employs a similar strategy to argue that lying is never justified. This is summarized nicely by James Rachels: "We could not will that it be a universal law that we should lie, because it would be self-defeating; people would quickly learn that they could not rely on what other people said, and so the lies would not be believed" (1993, p. 120). As with promising, the whole point in lying would be lost since every one would know one was lying. Thus, again, to universalize the practice of lying would be to destroy the point of lying.

Note that Kant's imperative does seem to be a central feature of commonsense morality. Often we try to appeal to people's moral sense by saying, 'What would the world be like if everyone acted like that?' For example, one might try to get a child to start to think in this way: if he were to steal another child's toy we might say, 'What if everyone behaved like you?' – the implication being that no one would actually have any toys of their own.

A further, famous formulation of the categorical imperative is this:

Act in such a way that you always treat humanity, whether in thine own person or in that of any other, never simply as a means, but always at the same time as an end. (Kant, 1948, p. 91)

This states that other humans are autonomous, rational moral agents and should be respected as such. So, according to this statement, institutions such as slavery are morally wrong because they involve treating humans as tools – purely as a means to the promotion of others' ends. Hence, it can be seen that it is not a criticism of a person's moral standards to say that he uses tools (hammers, screwdrivers and so on), but it is a criticism to say that a person uses other people. This formulation is especially relevant in the context of research on human beings. If the researcher has no moral regard for the research participants they are using them 'simply as a means' and are acting unethically.

Evidently, this formulation of Kant's imperative raises the distinction between categorical and hypothetical reasoning again. In reasoning categorically, a person thinks simply, 'I ought to do X'. But in using another person to further our own ends we are reasoning hypothetically: 'I desire X; to bring about X, I need S to do Y'. Let us now turn to some comments on Kant's approach before we move on to some criticisms of it.

Comments on Kantian theory

Kant's emphasis on the motives and intentions of the actor seems obviously correct. Evaluation of the intentions of the actor is of relevance to evaluating the morality of certain actions. Recall the example given earlier between the two people who make the donations to charity; we distinguish between the moral character of their actions. The one who gives to charity because it is the right thing to do is acting morally, but this is less obviously true of the person who does so because they are forced into it. The further relevance of intentions is evident in law: if a person performs an act intentionally, from premeditation, he is considered more culpable than a person who commits the same act unintentionally (note the distinction between murder and manslaughter).

Also, the distinction between acting in conformity with duty and acting out of respect for duty again seems to carry great plausibility. It is, furthermore, central to moral thought. Commonsense moral thought clearly distinguishes between a student nurse who makes an incontinent patient comfortable due to recognition of a moral duty to do so, and a student nurse who performs the same act solely to impress the senior nurse.

In addition, the point that moral theories should respect the central components in the commonsense theory seems to be one of great importance. It is plausible to think that commonsense moral thought will always be the tribunal or testing ground against which the deliverances of moral theories will be assessed. If a theorist claimed to have devised a moral theory which radically conflicted with the commonsense theory, would it be accepted? (It should be stressed, though, that this is not to say that, for Kant, moral theory should merely reflect ordinary moral thought: see e.g., Kant, 1948, p. 73.) Having made these observations about Kant's approach, let us turn to some criticisms.

Some criticisms

Throughout the exposition of Kant's theory, reference has been made to 'the commonsense theory' or to ordinary moral thought, and it has been said that this provides a starting point for Kant. But there are at least two difficulties which follow from reliance on commonsense moral theory. First, the commonsense view of moral matters which informed Kant's thought is one which existed in eighteenth-century Europe. Is it the case that the categorical imperative (or 'Golden Rule' as it is sometimes called) still occupies the central position in moral thinking which Kant claims for it (even if it did then)?

Second, even if it is accepted that commonsense moral thought has not substantially changed in bare essentials, the view there is an absolute prohibition against lying is in serious conflict with ordinary moral thought. Is it generally believed to be the case that one should never, under any circumstances tell a lie? Or are there exceptions? A common, critical response to Kant's view is presented by a case in which lying looks ethically justified. Thus for example if you are hiding an innocent, close friend of yours from some ruthless criminals who intend to kill that person, it would seem right to lie to the criminals if they were to ask you where your friend is. Although you tell a lie, by ordinary moral standards that would be justified because you save the life of the person. Yet, as we saw, lying is never justified for Kant. This seems very implausible. What the example shows is that, contrary to what Kant thinks, consequences can be morally relevant in assessing the morality of an act.

Also, contrary to Kant's intentions, it looks like it may be possible to devise a version of the categorical imperative in such a way that lying in some specific types of situation, may turn out to be justified. So, for example, suppose in deciding whether or not to lie to the criminals one's rule is formulated in this way: 'I will that it is right to lie when a murderer threatens to kill a close friend'. It looks like one can universalize this without it leading to the kind of problem that occurs if one universalizes a rule such as 'it is right to lie when it is to one's own advantage'. This is because it only applies in situations involving ruthless criminals, as opposed to all other kinds of situation.

A further criticism is that the theory is too rigid and therefore is inappropriate in the health care setting. There may well be situations in which it is justifiable to lie, as in the situation we have just described in which doing so will save someone's life or will protect them from serious harm. Here the duties to protect life and not to lie come in to conflict with no clear way evident about how to resolve the problem.

Moreover, as the last point illustrates Kantian theory leaves us with a problem if we have conflicting duties. For example, if it is always wrong to break a promise, how can one respond to a situation in which one has conflicting promises?

So although there are things of great importance in Kant's theory, it does not look adequate. Its inflexibility and its problems regarding situations when duties conflict mean that we need to look elsewhere. Also, in nursing, many nurses have been critical of Kantian approaches to ethics which they see as excessively rational and of neglecting more 'care orientated' considerations (but see Paley, 2002 for a defence). They complain that acting in the right way need not involve the kind of calculation required by the categorical imperative. In some situations, the morally right thing to do is simply to respond because one cares about others, not because one has worked out that that is what duty requires. We will return to discuss this alternative, care-based approach in a later chapter. We now turn to consider a theory which is an ancient one, being proposed first by Aristotle (384–322 BC). The theory has attracted much interest during the last 50 years or so, and is frequently referred to in the context of nursing ethics (for a thorough treatment of its application to nursing, see Armstrong, 2007).

Ethics of virtue

As mentioned, the third type of approach to moral thinking to be described here is virtue ethics. It has seemed plausible to many that an ethics of virtue will have particular relevance to nursing. This is because, it is said, nursing practice involves virtues such as kindness, honesty, care, benevolence, compassion, courage and loyalty. So it seems logical that if these are so important to nursing, so too must an approach to ethics in which they have a prominent place. The kinds of concerns to which the previous two theories seem vulnerable have also led many to embrace virtue ethics. But what is it? The description of it to be given now will begin by setting it in the nursing context.

In the context of nursing the view that some character traits will be possessed by a good nurse is a common one. For example we might agree that a good nurse will be caring, kind, honest, compassionate, benevolent, courageous and so on. But the idea of character traits in themselves seems a bit too broad. Being greedy, selfish or unscrupulous are also character traits and these would not be thought desirable in a good nurse. To distinguish character traits which are desirable in the good nurse from those which are not, the term favoured by virtue ethicists is that of virtues. So those character traits thought desirable can be classed as virtues, and those which one hopes to be absent in the good nurse we can call vices. The good nurse is a virtuous nurse who acts virtuously. If a novice nurse wants to know how to conduct herself or himself and respond to ethical challenges in nursing practice, he or she can be pointed in the direction of the virtuous nurse: watch and learn from how *she* deals with awkward problems in nursing practice. The good nurse thus manifests excellence in such practice; others that aspire to that level should try to learn to be like her, to develop the same set of virtues themselves. Put another way, the good nurse has developed these 'habits' (Aristotle, *Ethics*, 1955 edition, p. 55) of virtuous behaviour, the aspiring novice nurse should try to acquire and cultivate these too.

To give an example to try to illustrate the difference between this approach and the previous two, consider a nurse who is asked a question by a patient. The patient's prognosis is very poor, but the patient does not yet know this, although she has been ill for over a year, being treated for a serious condition. The patient is only 8 years old and her parents have just been told their daughter's condition is no longer treatable and that she is likely to die within a matter of months. The parents state that they want to give this bad news to their daughter themselves, but will need a few moments, perhaps an hour, to compose themselves sufficiently to be able to break the awful news to their child. It is agreed amongst the health care team that they will respect the wishes of the parents in this case.

Having come from the meeting with the parents, and aware of the parents' plan, a nurse is called by the patient. The patient asks when will she start to get better.

We know from the description of duty-based ethics that a nurse whose practice is informed by this, is not permitted to lie. She will apply the categorical imperative to determine what moral duty requires, and then respond accordingly. The Utilitarian will calculate which responses generate the best overall consequences – which will maximize overall happiness – and then respond accordingly. Note that in each of these descriptions, some calculation is required in order to determine the right moral response. If the calculation is done competently, the morally right response results.

But what of the virtuous nurse, how would she respond? What we can expect is that such a nurse brings appropriate virtues to bear on the situation. These can be expected to include virtues of benevolence, respect, compassion, and perhaps courage. The last virtue might be necessary if the nurse thinks it right to be truthful to the patient at that time, in spite of what the parents have said. If the nurse is truthful, one can say she acted compassionately, with respect for the patient, and also courageously for the reason just noted.

To explain this a little. It is part of the concept of virtue ethics that the virtuous person develops the habit of being virtuous. So, to illustrate, imagine that one seeks to develop the virtue of temperance. This is not abstinence, but moderation – somewhere between abstinence and incontinence (lack of control of one's drinking alcohol). Suppose one is in the habit of drinking heavily each evening. Clearly one lacks the virtue of temperance. In seeking to acquire it one might need to implement a strategy for controlling one's desire for alcohol, since one is currently in the habit of consuming large amounts of it each night. The suggested strategy might include doing some other kinds of activity which distract one from the temptation to drink; this might be evening classes, exercise, taking one's children out or studying. In the early stages one feels this to be something of a struggle, the desire for alcohol competes with the desire for temperance. Eventually if one succeeds in the struggle, not drinking excessively every night becomes a habit, one acquires the virtue of temperance.

A similar story can be told in relation to virtues more salient to contemporary nursing practice. One might enter nursing already equipped with the relevant virtues, thus it is apparently in one's nature to be kind, sensitive, caring, courageous and so on. But if not, the process of becoming a good nurse involves acquiring the relevant virtues, at first consciously (as in the 'temperance' example) but then, one hopes, it becomes habitual to behave virtuously.

Some situations may be so complicated, though, that the virtuous habits we have are insufficient to deal with the complexity of the situation. There, more care may be needed in developing the virtuous response to the situation. So it should not be thought that the virtuous nurse unreflectively knows which action is called for by the virtues.

We began this exposition of virtue-based ethics by posing a question about the characteristics of the good nurse. As was pointed out, a distinctive feature of virtue ethics is its focus on character rather than acts ('what would a good person do?' 'What should I do?' As opposed to 'what is the right thing to do?). It was then pointed out that the virtues that might plausibly be possessed by the good nurse were those of care, compassion, benevolence, courage, amongst others. The suggestion then is that novice nurses, in working with a good nurse, one whose practice exemplifies these virtues, if they are capable of doing so, will gradually acquire these virtues. At first this might involve a kind of 'consciously executed' learning process (as in the 'temperance' example) but gradually acting virtuously will become ingrained and habitual.

Although we have explicated virtue ethics with reference solely to nursing, it was of course originally proposed as a general ethical theory by Aristotle. His claims concern the good *person* as opposed to the good nurse. Hence his enquiry tries to set out the virtues that a good person would possess and would manifest in their leading a good life. In his view virtues are always to be found between extremes. His thought is that extremes are to be avoided. Thus the virtue of courage is a mean between the extremes of recklessness and cowardice. The virtue of temperance is that between extremes of intemperance and abstinence. With regard to care (though I do not think this is a virtue he discusses) this could be viewed as a mean between the extremes of callousness and 'over involvement'.

It might be thought that the idea of the 'mean' works less well in relation to a virtue such as honesty. Can we conceive of 'extreme honesty' as a bad thing, a vice? To see that it might be, consider a person who tells the truth on all occasions, irrespective of the circumstances. So instead of telling a proud new parent that their baby is indeed beautiful, she says it looks ugly. Instead of praising the efforts of a young child when he clumsily attempts to tie his shoelaces, one points out that the child has failed again. It seems plain that to be truthful on *all* occasions would be a moral flaw, not a virtue. So even in the case of honesty, the suggestion that this is a mean between extremes seems plausible.

So we have some idea of what a virtue is: it is a disposition to act virtuously. But what is the connection between possession of virtues and being a good person? To try to illustrate this, we saw above that it is possible to identify some of the characteristics of a good nurse, and to describe these in terms of the virtues. As mentioned, such a nurse might be caring, kind, compassionate, courageous and so on. A similar suggestion can be made when trying to identify the characteristics of a good person. Such a person, it seems reasonable to claim, would be a virtuous one (Aristotle *Ethics*, p. 64). They would be kind, sensitive, courageous, loyal, honest, temperate, compassionate, conscientious, and so on. Suppose you are applying for a job and you approach someone to give you the best reference you can think of. You would be hoping that the description of you would include at least a few of those virtues we have just listed.

So the good person, then, is a virtuous one. One cannot simply become virtuous overnight. One must, instead, cultivate virtuous habits as described above. Part of this, will be honing the kinds of dimensions of the moral life mentioned in Chapter 1. These were moral sensitivity, perception and imagination.

Our exposition of virtue-based ethics began with a discussion of the idea of the good nurse. We then turned to discuss virtue ethics in its more general application in terms of the good person. Before moving on to some comments on and criticisms of the virtue-based approach, a word is needed on the relationship between the 'role virtues' which inform the practice of the good nurse, and the virtues more generally – those possessed by the good person.

Suppose these come into conflict. What should one do? It is plausible to think that the virtues of the good person, should prevail in such a conflict. Hence what would matter most would be the virtues the nurse possesses as a virtuous *person*. To see this, consider a virtue which used to be held prominently in nursing ethics, obedience to authority, in particular the authority of senior nurses and medical staff (Dock, 1900). Suppose a nurse witnesses mistreatment of a patient by a senior nurse or doctor. If obedience really is a virtue in nursing, the nurse, it seems, would be obliged to stay silent about this if instructed to do so by the senior figure. Such a nurse would have a conflict between the 'role' virtues of a nurse and the more general virtues of the good person. It seems implausible to think that a virtue theory would require the nurse to stay within the role virtues and suppress what virtue requires from her as a virtuous person.

Comments and criticisms

The last discussion highlights one problem of virtue ethics, which is that of their variance across historical periods and across cultures. Obedience may have been a key virtue of the nurse, but surely it is not any longer. The NMC Code (2008) makes plain that protection of patients is more important than obedience to authority figures ('You must make the care of people your first concern'). This variance leads to uncertainty in relation to the virtues. A nurse might wonder whether she should bother to cultivate a particular virtue in case by the time she acquires it, it is considered unsuitable for a nurse to possess it. Similarly, the novice nurse might disagree with the way in which an experienced nurse, held to be a role model, deals with patients. The novice nurse might think her scepticism is justified since the character traits called virtues are transient over time and culturally variant.

A second common criticism is that it seems difficult to respond adequately to situations in which virtues conflict. In the example given above of the 8-year-old patient whose parents want to tell her themselves that she will not be getting better; relevant virtues include compassion, respect, benevolence, courage, honesty. Suppose the nurse decided to be truthful to the patient, against the wishes of the parents. This decision may be driven by virtues of respect, honesty and courage and benevolence. But what if a different nurse judged benevolence to guide her to keeping the information from the patient? She might explain such a decision by saying that the most benevolent course of action would be to let the parents break the bad news. And further, that respect for the parents is a key consideration. The courage involved lies in the courage to omit to tell the truth to the patient in the knowledge that the parents will do so later. So there looks to be a problem in deciding which virtues to manifest the most when a moral problem arises, this is because both acts can seem virtuous.

This last problem raises a third concern. The other two theories we have considered seem able to offer direction if one is wondering how to respond to a moral problem. For the Utilitarian we should try to maximize utility, for the deontologist we should do what duty requires, and we can find out what this is by invoking the categorical imperative. But it seems that the most the virtue theorist can offer is to tell us to act as a virtuous person would act, or to 'be virtuous'. This does not seem much help. Even if one eventually acquires all the attributes of the virtuous nurse, it will take time to do so. And one will encounter moral problems to deal with throughout that time. So more moral guidance is needed than simply 'be virtuous'.

In spite of these three problems with the approach, there is something of merit in it. The emphasis on moral character seems important. We do think there is more to morality than simply the performance of the right actions. We would expect such actions to be done from the right motives, for example from respect or honesty or kindness. And as patients we would hope that the nurses caring for us are genuinely disposed to be good, to do their best for us. They are not simply acting out a role, a pretence of caring. Also, the kinds of phenomena mentioned in Chapter 1 concerning moral awareness, perception and imagination are aspects of the moral life which have received particular emphasis in virtue ethics, and for the reasons given in Chapter 1, seem important aspects of morally sensitive nursing practice.

Moreover, one can identify close relations between the moral obligations set out in the four principles and corresponding virtues (Beauchamp and Childress, 2009, p. 45). So corresponding to the principles of beneficence, non-maleficence and justice, are virtues of benevolence, non-malevolence and fairness. The virtue of respect would correspond to many of the dimensions featured within the principle of respect for autonomy. Indeed some virtue theorists incorporate directives akin to moral rules – so-called 'v-rules' (Hursthouse, 1999) which seem close to the principles. Thus, as with Utilitarianism, there is scope within virtue theory for a distinction between 'act' and 'rule' versions of the theory. In an act version each situation is responded to in its own right. But in a rule version certain virtue-rules are identified. It is plausible to think of the four principles as playing such a role, especially if supplemented with the emphasis on moral character and perception.

So we have seen basic introductions to the four levels of moral reasoning identified at the start of the chapter. And we have seen in our discussions of three moral theories that none is impervious to criticism. What we need to do now is to try to gain some idea of how these levels are related.

How are the four levels related?

In early editions of Beauchamp and Childress's book (*Principles of Biomedical Ethics*) the relationship between the levels was presented in such way that the most general level – that of moral theories – ultimately provided support for the less general levels – levels one, two and three. Thus in Rule Utilitarianism level-one judgements would be justified by appeal to level-two rules, the justification for these being the level-four theory, Utilitarianism. Such a Rule Utilitarian omits level-three principles and simply moves from level-one judgements, to level-two rules to level four. Alternatively, the Rule Utilitarian might consider that level-three principles provide a justification for level-two rules. Such a theorist, thus, holds that judgements are justified by rules, which in turn are justified by principles, which in turn are justified due to the fact that their application serves to maximize utility.

Evidently, the 'direction' of justification here goes from the particular judgement to the general rule, principle or theory. So a decision to tell the truth would be justified by a moral rule (veracity) which would be justified in turn by a moral principle (respect for autonomy) and the justification for this would lie in the moral theory – in the truth-telling example we are discussing, that of Utilitarianism.

A difficulty with this kind of approach is that, as we have seen, the first two moral theories we considered seem vulnerable to serious objection. So any attempt at justification of particular moral judgements which ultimately rested on the credibility of the theory would be bound to fail. This is because such a foundation would be inherently shaky due to the flaws in the moral theory.

This is the case also with reference to virtue theory. As seen, ultimately, the virtue theorist relies on our ability to do what the virtuous person would do. But this seems unhelpful and vague. This is the case even though, as we have seen, some aspects of virtue theory are important, and there seem close connections between some virtues and the kinds of moral values captured in the four principles.

So if the relationship between the levels of the framework is *not* one in which there are ascending levels of justification, what is the relationship between them? In the first edition of this book, it was argued that the level at which the principles feature is the most important of the four levels which Beauchamp and Childress identify. We will rehearse that case again shortly, but first here it is important to indicate how Beauchamp and Childress themselves deal with this problem.

They propose what they call a 'coherence theory' or equivalently a 'reflective equilibrium' model (2009, p. 381). In this, there are no ultimate foundations which support moral judgements, but there are some very widely agreed sets of values. These can be found to be present in all moral theories, and in commonsense approaches to moral problems; that is, in the approaches which we all take in our daily interactions with one another. The idea is that by reflecting on moral values present within commonsense morality, and on those presented by other perspectives, one can arrive at a system of defensible moral judgements. These would reflect a broad consensus.

Of course to say this is not necessarily to equate moral rightness or wrongness with consensus. A consensus might be flawed. For example, suppose a consensus view was that women should not be given the vote, or as at present, that it is morally permissible to eat meat from animals. It would not follow necessarily that these views would have the status of unchallengeable moral truths. If they can be shown to conflict with other moral beliefs, which are also given great weight, then the possibility of revision arises. And in the case of the first example that is what happened of course. The view that women be denied the vote was seen to conflict with the view that humans have equal rights, or that they should be treated with equal respect. The example also shows that such changes in the moral landscape will occur, but that the change in consensus may be preceded by a period of vigorous debate in which the position taken to constitute current consensus is disputed by challengers and defended by others. Also, of course some disputes may prove not to be resolvable to the satisfaction of all. The presence of a consensus is consistent with the presence of vigorous opponents of aspects of it. The current, ongoing debate in the UK about the legalization of abortion is a good example of this. A consensus exists to the effect that abortion, in some circumstances, is permissible. But there are vocal opponents of that consensus.

So this is the kind of approach Beauchamp and Childress present as being more plausible than approaches in which the theories provide an unshakeable moral foundation for principles, rules and judgements. The approach recognizes the complexity of the moral sphere and tries to incorporate all relevant moral considerations. Thus the merits of the various moral theories will be represented in the 'coherence' approach. In other words appeals to consequences, duties, virtues, rights and care will all have force. But appeals to them will not be compelling. To my mind this coherence view reinforces the importance that can be attached to the moral principles. For they provide key reference points in commonsense morality and so provide a helpful focus for moral thinking and decision-making. This line of argument will be developed further in the next section.

Arguments for the priority of moral principles

In this section it will be contended that it is level three of Beauchamp and Childress's framework for moral reasoning, as opposed to its other levels, which is the most relevant to moral deliberation in nursing ethics, and the following arguments in support of that claim are offered.

First, it is plausible that level three is of greater moral importance than levels one and two. This is due simply to the fact the principles are more general than the rules and judgements in levels one and two. The level-three principles provide a justification for the level-two rules and, derivatively, for level-one judgements. This is illustrated by the point that a decision to tell the truth can be justified by the veracity rule which in turn is justified in terms of the principle of respect for autonomy.

Second, of the three level-four moral theories identified earlier, two proved divisible into act and rule variations. Thus we identified Act

Utilitarianism and Rule Utilitarianism, and act and rule versions of virtue theory. The 'Act' variations respond, case by case, to particular situations. They base their decisions about how to act on the characteristics of each particular situation as opposed to articulating general principles of the kind developed by Beauchamp and Childress.

However, at least two serious criticisms can be levelled at approaches which reject wholesale the adoption of general principles or rules which apply to relevantly similar sets of circumstances. To illustrate the problems with approaches which focus just on particular acts and which neglect the development of moral rules or principles, suppose it is claimed by someone supporting such an approach, that an act of type A is morally right in a circumstance (situation) of type C. It is plain that theorists who make such a judgement must be committed to the view that acts of type A are morally right in all other circumstances (situations) of type C (cf. Hare, 1981). For example, suppose acts of type A are acts of truth-telling, and circumstances of type C concern those in which a competent person requests information concerning his medical condition. It seems that Act Utilitarianism and Deontology must commit one to acting in the same way in all relevantly similar sets of circumstances. If act A maximizes utility in one instance of C, surely it must do so in all instances of C. Similarly, when the position of the Deontologist is considered: if it is one's duty to tell the truth in one instance of circumstances of type C, it follows that it is one's duty to do so in all circumstances of type C. The same must be true of an act version of virtue theory.

So, the idea that 'Act' approaches can coherently claim to be simply considering one situation at a time is dubious. Decisions concerning what is right or wrong in one instance of a type of circumstance imply that the act theorists are obliged to act in the same types of ways in relevantly similar types of circumstances.

Further, against the 'Act' approaches their approach is of extremely limited use in practice. This follows since it requires persons to consider each situation anew, and to apply either the principle of utility or the categorical imperative to it, or to respond virtuously to it. Seedhouse (1988, p. 94) points out that although many situations have aspects unique to them, it is possible to identify morally relevant similarities between situations. And, he suggests that the identification of common characteristics of types of situations can help to formulate general rules which can be applied in relevantly similar cases. Adoption of such rules (or principles) facilitates consistency in moral thinking, and, importantly, is intimately connected with fairness in the making of moral decisions. As noted earlier, put crudely, the principle of justice demands that at least that equals be treated equally. Plausibly, this requires that we make consistent moral judgements in relevantly similar cases; and this in turn appears to require that some assessment is made to the effect that two situations are indeed relevantly similar or are not relevantly similar. This appears to conflict with the general approach to moral decision-making canvassed in the 'Act' approaches considered here.

The arguments presented so far in this section suggest that of the level-four theories identified above (Act Utilitarianism, Rule Utilitarianism, Deontology, Rule Virtue theory and Act Virtue Theory), all 'Act' versions are vulnerable to serious objection.

Consider the following argument which is supposed to show that Rule Utilitarianism is less adequate than the four level-three principles when it comes to moral decision-making – specifically in nursing practice (virtue theory will be considered separately below).

As discussed earlier in this chapter, Utilitarianism asserts that the rightness or the wrongness of an action depends solely upon its outcome. From the perspective of a duty-based theory, on the other hand, the rightness or the wrongness of an act is wholly independent of its consequences; what matters is that the actor acts out of respect for moral duty. But whilst each theory captures something of importance, neither is adequate on its own. When faced with a moral problem, one needs to consider both what it is one's duty to do, and what the consequences of one's actions are likely to be. This is especially the case in relation to moral problems faced by nurses. Minimally, nurses are obliged to consider what is their duty when faced with particular moral problems in nursing practice – both moral and professional duty. But, further, it is plausible to hold that nurses are also obliged to consider the consequences of their decisions about moral matters. For example, suppose a nurse undertakes a particular action, say, pressing a fire alarm. Suppose further that this is done out of respect for duty: the nurse believes there to be a fire on the ward, and so presses the alarm. The relevant professional duties here are those stated in the clause of the NMC Code according to which the nurse must 'protect the health and well being of those in your care' (2008); and the relevant moral duties are those referred to by the principles of beneficence and non-maleficence. Evidently, the nurse presses the alarm because a consequence of not doing so is a high probability of harm to others. Plausibly, then, the nurse is compelled to act out of respect for duty due to the necessity of acting in accord with the clauses in the NMC Code, and due to the necessary connection between nursing actions and morality;

and is compelled to consider the consequences of his or her actions in evaluating how to put duty into effect (how to make it the case that patients are protected from harm). So, in moral decision-making in the nursing context it is evident that it is necessary to consider both the consequences of one's actions and what it is one's duty to do and that both are relevant to the moral appraisal of the action. Indeed, further, it could be suggested that it is morally reprehensible not to consider the consequences of one's actions when making moral decisions.

So, it is being claimed here that it is necessary for nurses to consider both duties and consequences in their moral decision-making and that both consequences and duties are relevant to the moral rightness or wrongness of an action. Another example to lend support to this point is the following: consider a psychiatric nurse who agrees to a request by a patient to leave the ward, and that the nurse has good grounds to believe that the patient is sufficiently mentally competent, and well enough to do so without coming to any harm. From the moral perspective, the nurse acts out of consideration for the principle of respect for autonomy, and makes no attempt to physically prevent the patient from leaving the ward (perhaps by invoking the holding power ascribed to nurses under the Mental Health Act, 1983, as amended 2007). Suppose, further, that it then transpires that the patient commits suicide and that the nurse is called upon to account for her decision. The nurse might argue that her decision was made to respect the wishes of a competent person and was grounded in respect for autonomy. Even if the nurse acts in that way (placing respect for autonomy over principle of non-maleficence), the nurse should and would consider the consequences of the action. An investigating coroner might reasonably put to the nurse the question, 'Did you consider the possibility that the patient might take his or her own life?' The nurse, if professionally and morally competent, must have an answer to this question. Whether the nurse answers 'yes' or 'no' – and, conceivably, either of these answers may be acceptable depending upon the circumstances – it would be barely coherent for the nurse to make both of the following claims: (a) that she was acting professionally and morally, and (b) that she omitted to consider the consequences of her decision to agree to the patient's competently expressed wish to leave the ward. This shows that consequences are morally relevant (which is not to say, of course, that only consequences are morally relevant).

These considerations strongly suggest that in moral deliberations about nursing practice, it is necessary to consider both what is one's duty and to consider the consequences of one's actions.

It seems fair to conclude, then, that at level four of Beauchamp and Childress's moral framework, we should not retain an exclusive commitment either to Utilitarianism or to a Kantian duty-based morality but, rather, adopt the general stance in our moral decision-making that it is morally best to consider both consequences and duties since each are relevant to the moral justification of acts.

The criticisms just made have been directed at Utilitarian and duty-based approaches, but we temporarily set virtue theory aside. The reason is that it is, of course, plausible that the actions of nurses should stem from and should manifest appropriate virtues. But having said this, two qualifications are needed.

Here is the first, the criticism of 'act' approaches given above shows that a rule version of virtue theory is the more plausible. And, as proposed in the discussion of virtue theory above, there is a close concordance between the four principles and virtues such as benevolence, respect, non-malevolence and fairness. Moreover, Chapter 1 endorsed the 'moral psychology' associated with virtue ethics regarding awareness, perception and imagination. So it is accepted that it is a good thing if nurses act virtuously in accord with the virtues captured in the principles. In other words, if a nurse applies the principles virtuously that is not to be discouraged. But it is too much to *require* that nurses do this. Nor would it make much sense to do so (imagine: 'you must be virtuous in your dealings with patients').

But, by contrast, it is of course reasonable to *require* nurses to practice in accord with the four principles. They should respect patients' autonomy, promote their well-being, not harm them and treat them fairly. In contrast to the virtues it is indeed reasonable to require that practice manifests these moral values. There may be situations when it is not possible to respect autonomy, or perhaps even to promote well-being of patients. But in such situations a reason must be given to explain why not (such as 'the patient lacks autonomy', 'the patient's death is imminent' and so on).

In the light of the above arguments concerning level four of the framework, it will be proposed here that it is level three – that relating to moral principles – which is the most important level for our purposes. This is due to the following five reasons:

1. In contrast to the level-four theories, the level-three principles are easily applicable to the vast majority of moral problems faced by nurses. The principles provide a structure for the moral intuitions brought to moral problems by nurses. Consequently, consideration of

moral problems through the lens of level-three principles ensures that practitioners consider the situation from a number of perspectives – the perspective of each principle.

2. Second, overemphasis of the importance of level-four theories can foster the view that there are clear solutions to moral problems: simply act in such a way as to maximize utility; or simply apply the categorical imperative, or do what the virtuous nurse would do. But this is too simplistic and unhelpful. Moral problems do not lend themselves to readily available answers thrown up by moral theories. It is surely preferable to consider the situation from a number of perspectives – those of the principles – rather than attempt to evaluate which course of action is morally correct. Of course, a decision does have to be made; but it would seem preferable that such a decision emerges from consideration of various ways of viewing the situation, rather than, simply, implementing a particular level-four theory.

3. Further, from the author's experience of teaching nurses, it is evident that they themselves think the principles of level three easier to apply and more relevant to practice than the level-four theories. Given introductory outlines of the four principles, nurses begin to structure their moral thinking by reference to them. This kind of teaching can be deployed to foster the virtues in nursing too. As nurses begin to think and notice the moral dimension of practice, with good role models and some effort, they can learn how to be good nurses. As explained above, this minimally must include thinking about moral problems in terms of the four principles and manifesting this thinking in terms of ethical responses to problems.

4. Fourthly, as will be shown later, moral thinking at the level of principles does allow one to develop a coherent, well-motivated strategy by which to help to try to resolve moral dilemmas – given that these result from clashes between principles themselves.

5. Fifthly, nurses are bound by the professional obligations set out in the NMC Code to respect the individuality of patients and it is reasonable to interpret this, if only in part, in terms of respecting their autonomy. It is evident (see Chapter 3) that the principles of level three of the framework underlie many clauses in the NMC Code. So, plausibly, whether the ultimate moral justification for the principles is grounded in Utilitarian, duty-based or virtuous considerations, nurses are required to engage in moral thinking at the level of principles simply to fulfil their professional obligations.

Thus far, I have been relatively uncritical of the principle-based approach to nursing ethics. But there are at least two important areas of controversy which need to be mentioned. A first question concerns the weighting of the four principles which we have referred to so far. Are they each to be accorded the same moral 'weight', so to speak, so that in a conflict between moral principles we should be paralysed, and unsure how to act? Or, are some principles more weighty than others, so that in a conflict we may judge which principle carries most weight and hence which obligations are the more pressing? This question is one to be discussed in the next chapter following further consideration of the four principles. A second question is much more radical – this casts doubt on the legitimacy of the principle-based approach as a whole and champions an alternative, care-based approach to nursing ethics. Discussion of that debate is postponed until Chapter 5.

Conclusion

A considerable amount of work has been done in this chapter. We have identified four different levels of thinking about moral matters and sought to explain each of them: judgements, rules, principles and theories. Towards the close of the chapter arguments were presented to show that of the four levels of moral thinking identified, it is the level of principles which is the most important for our purposes. What needs to be done now, then, is to say much more about each principle and this task is to be undertaken in the next chapter.

Chapter 3

The Four Principles: Respect for Autonomy, Beneficence, Non-maleficence and Justice

In this chapter we look in more depth each of the four principles defined briefly in the previous chapter. Also, we try to develop a controversial version of the principle-based approach, one which accords greatest weight to the principle of respect for autonomy. This brings some advantages in terms of moral decision-making and clarity, but as will be seen there are costs too. The chapter closes by setting out the close relationship between the clauses in the NMC Code (2008; see Appendix) and the four principles described in the chapter.

The principle of respect for autonomy

The term 'autonomy' derives from a Greek word meaning 'self-governing' (Beauchamp and Childress, 2009, p. 99). This gives some indication of what it means in the health care context. To say that a person has autonomy, or equivalently, is autonomous, is to say that they have the capacity for self-government. In other words, they are capable of making their own decisions about matters which concern their own life.

This is simply a description of what is involved in a person's having the capacity to be autonomous. A person is autonomous if they are self-governing, where this involves the ability to make decisions about one's life. Such decisions can be trivial, such as a decision about which kind of chocolate bar to eat at lunch time; and they can be of the utmost seriousness, such as a decision to donate a kidney to a living relative, or to forego life-prolonging medical treatment.

The *moral principle* of respect for autonomy concerns obligations to respect the kinds of choices just mentioned – those that are produced by autonomous people. For obvious reasons, this can be regarded as a 'passive' aspect of the moral principle; it simply states an obligation to respect the choices of others. But respect for autonomy has a more demanding 'active' aspect to it too. This involves information giving. The rationale for this is easy to see. We need information to make informed, and thus autonomous, choices. If we have only incomplete information, then our ability to make genuine choices is impaired. In other words, our ability to 'self-govern' is reduced.

Note that to bombard a patient with so much information that they feel baffled is not to respect their autonomy. To overwhelm a patient with information – even if the information is relevant to the patient – is not to respect that patient's autonomy. For overwhelming a patient with information is not conducive to their ability to self-govern. For the same reason, providing a patient with relevant information, but in terminology they cannot understand, is also to fail to respect autonomy.

The obligations referred to by this principle are highlighted by many commentators (Gillon, 1985; Beauchamp and Childress, 2009). And some have suggested that the principle of respect for autonomy is the most fundamental of all moral principles (cf. Mill, 1859; Benjamin and Curtis, 1986; Gillon, 2003). In the context of nursing, this would entail that nurses should give highest regard to their obligations to respect the autonomy of their patients. Further, if an autonomous decision made by a patient is to be overruled by others, then the burden of justification lies with those who would seek to overrule it.

An example in which we might want to overrule a patient's autonomous decision is a case where an informal patient (one not detained compulsorily under a section of the Mental Health Act) on a mental health ward makes a decision to leave the ward. A paper in the journal *Open Mind* (anon., 1991, pp. 7–10) is entitled 'Free to leave at any time?': the clear implication of the title is that although informal patients might *legally* be free to leave at any time, in practice that often turns out not to be the case. The writers of the article claim that almost 8,000 requests to leave hospital made by informal clients in the year 1988–89 were refused. If those requests were made by autonomous patients, who were competent to make the decision, then such refusals indicate violations of the principle of respect for autonomy (see also Lutzen, 1998 and O'Brien and Golding, 2003 on this topic). To say this is not (yet) to say that such transgressions of the principle of respect for autonomy were unjustified. It is impossible to know this without further information regarding the instances. Nonetheless, the writers of the article clearly imply that these were unjustified breaches of respect for patient autonomy in their view.

What needs to be considered now is just what it is that is so special about respecting autonomy that it should occupy such a prominent place in nursing and health care ethics.

Why autonomy?

As we have noted, many theorists writing in the area of health care ethics attach great importance to the principle of respect for autonomy. It might be worth considering why autonomy should be accorded such status – why should it be thought that overruling autonomy requires justification? Much hinges on this question since the reasons to be offered here contribute to a general claim that the obligations referred to by the principle of respect for autonomy are the most important of all the obligations referred to by the four principles.

First, it can be noted that there is something slightly insulting about someone whom one meets and who simply presumes that one is not autonomous. Perhaps the person treats you like a small child, making decisions on your behalf which you are perfectly able to make yourself. Such a person is behaving paternalistically and one might justifiably feel offended at this. If we as autonomous individuals object to being patronized, and if we feel uncomfortable when this happens, we may plausibly conclude that other people object to being patronized just as we do to it. We infer from what happens in our own case and generalize it to others: if we were in their position we would object to being patronized. When someone patronizes us they are not respecting our autonomy, and many of us object to being treated in that way.

To try to express the same point in different terms, failing to respect the autonomy of another person is to place limits on their life choices. Since part of our development as people involves our making choices, and making mistakes, someone who prevents us from so doing is restricting our 'self-project', where this is our pursuance of the kind of life we want to lead, and the kind of person we want to become – our 'life plan' to put it grandly. So to fail to respect autonomy is indeed to do something very significant since it obstructs the pursuance of a life plan. And what seems objectionable about this is that it is surely up to us to decide what kind of person we want to become, what kind of plans we want to pursue.

Second, it seems clear that autonomy is regarded as something of value at least in Western cultures, but perhaps also in all cultures. Beauchamp and Childress claim the values captured in the four principles are universal – found in all cultures at all times (2009, p. 381). It is considered both desirable and psychologically healthy to be able to make up one's own mind, to be independent, and to be assertive when necessary (this, presumably, explains why some people attend so-called assertiveness training courses). Further, it is considered undesirable to be excessively passive and unassertive. In short, it appears that we value independence, and regard excess passivity and compliance with the wishes of others as undesirable and perhaps even psychologically unhealthy. This supports the idea that it is regarded as both desirable and healthy to be autonomous.

In amplification of this last point, think of the following situation. You have applied for a job and you ask a friend to provide your prospective employer with a reference. Your friend offers you a choice of two references. The first states that you are able to think for yourself and use your initiative; the second states that you cannot think for yourself and that you lack initiative. Which reference would you prefer your friend to send? Presumably, none of us would wish the second reference to be sent.

Third, it is plausible to claim that the whole notion of morality is dependent upon regarding other people as autonomous agents – as persons who are responsible for their actions. A person can only act morally if they do so intentionally and not, say, whilst they are under hypnosis. So, if it is true that it is only possible to act morally if one is an autonomous person, this indicates how central the notion of autonomy is to morality. (Note how, in law, people are punished more severely if their crime is premeditated.)

Fourth, if one considers which crimes are regarded as the most grave, the worst that one person can do to another, these include murder, assault and theft. Analysis of why this is the case shows that all these actions involve serious violations of respect for autonomy. To murder someone is to thwart a lifetime of future autonomous actions and choices; to assault a person is to override that person's autonomous wish to decide what should happen to her body; and, to steal from a person is to remove the possibility of that person autonomously deciding what to do with whatever is stolen (see also Singer, 1993, p. 99, on this topic). The proposed seriousness in morality of violations of autonomy is mirrored in law.

Consideration of punishments throws into relief the weight attached to respecting autonomy in our dealings with each other. To see this, consider that the most serious punishments which are given to people all involve curtailment of their autonomy. The most severe obviously is capital punishment. This curtails the autonomy of the offender wholesale. Imprisonment also is a curtailment of autonomy. If one is in prison one cannot enact one's autonomously chosen plans: one can't go wherever one chooses, meet one's friends and relatives, eat, drink and sleep as one chooses and so on. If one is fined, one can't spend that money in the way one would have chosen to. So it is evident that punishments are punishments because of the way they limit the autonomy of the offender.

Further, and fifth, it can be pointed out that the point of many interventions by health care professionals is to enhance the ability of patients to exercise their autonomy (cf. Seedhouse, 1988; Nordenfelt, 1995). For example, in the Adult Nursing context, suppose that a person needs to be admitted to hospital as a result of a badly broken leg. The person is able to make autonomous decisions, but, due to the broken leg, is unable to put them into effect. The role of the health care team, here, is plainly to repair the relevant parts of the person's body so that the person is again able to act upon autonomous decisions. Similar examples can be constructed concerning other conditions – say, peritonitis – and relating to other kinds of nursing (e.g., paediatric nursing and mental health nursing).

It can be added, also, on this point that the NMC Code (2004, clause 3.2 'You must respect patients' and clients' autonomy') strongly indicates that it is the duty of the nurse to respect and or 'foster' the autonomy of patients and clients. Hence, nursing actions which induce avoidable dependence on health care professionals would contravene the clause just referred to. Thus, actions such as feeding and dressing persons who can perform such tasks themselves, and who would prefer to do so themselves, may conflict with the duties set out in the previous NMC Code. This point is especially pertinent in the context of working with persons who have learning disabilities, and in the nursing care of older persons. It is easy to assume it to be necessary to perform the self-care of such people without really trying to determine whether or not they would prefer to do it themselves. To act in that way is to cultivate dependence on nursing staff and to omit to respect the autonomy of the person. The same points are expressed slightly differently in the NMC Code 2008, but they are still there. Thus for example it is stated 'You must listen to the people in your care and respond to their concerns and preferences' and 'You must support people in caring for themselves to improve and maintain their health' and lastly, 'You must recognise and respect the contribution that people make to their own care and wellbeing' (NMC, 2008).

Also, the importance attached to autonomy is reflected in law. Individuals are free to decide to reject even life-saving treatment. As Mason and McCall Smith state, 'Non-consensual medical treatment entitles the patient to sue for damages for the battery which is committed' (1994, p. 234). The above reasons, taken together, seem to indicate the enormous importance of the principle of respect for autonomy.

It might be objected that there are certain situations in nursing where it is not possible to foster or develop the autonomy of patients. Perhaps contexts such as the nursing of dying patients might be thought to throw up such examples. But even here a plausible response to such an objection can be offered. It can be argued that patients who are dying should be enabled to make known any views they have concerning their death, and that these should be respected. Such views might concern issues such as resuscitation, organ donation, which relatives they would like to be informed, which religious figures sent for, and so on. Fostering the autonomy of dying patients, therefore, can be claimed to involve creating a context in which they are able to express their own views concerning their own death. Such persons would then be enabled to die their own deaths, so to speak, and not die in the way others think best for them (see Woods, 2007).

It is worth drawing attention now to an idea which will be drawn upon later (Chapters 6 and 7), this is the idea of what we will term a 'life plan' (van Hooft, 1995). The idea here is that each of us in our minds has some fairly crude picture about the kind of life we wish to lead, and the way in which what we are currently doing contributes, or fails to contribute, to this. So, to take a simple example, suppose it is part one's life plan to work and to have a family that one is able to spend time with, and moreover to be able meet the conditions that are necessary for this. This is likely to include having some kind of income, some time to spend with one's family, enough money for essential needs such as food, warmth, shelter and safety and so on. Of course, someone else might have a completely different life plan, for example, rather than have their own family they may plan to spend their life in pursuit of their religious belief. Obviously, only autonomous people can have such plans. So the relationship between the idea of a life plan and that of autonomy is obvious. Also we can relate the idea of a life plan to the points made earlier regarding the importance of autonomy. Thus health care is important since it helps us to return to pursue our life plan after we have fallen ill. If we are very seriously ill we might have to revise our life plan. Punishments are punishments because they disrupt a life plan. As explained above, if one is in prison one can't be with one's family, choose with whom to socialize, choose when to go for a walk, and so on. Thus there is clearly an intimate connection between this idea of a life plan and the capacity to be autonomous. As mentioned this is an idea which we will return to in later chapters.

(It should be said that the case presented here in favour of respect for autonomy leads on to some much deeper discussions regarding the ultimate foundations, if any, of morality and also the nature of persons. It is not appropriate for us to pursue such discussions here but those interested might look at Mulhall and Swift's book *Liberals and Communitarians* (published by Blackwell, 1992) which provides a useful way into some of the issues underlying our discussion of autonomy.)

So far, the discussion has been concerned with what autonomy is, and also why it is so important to respect it. But it is also clear that there are occasions when it is not possible to respect a person's autonomy. A patient may have a very severe learning disability, or be in the acute phase of a mental health problem, or be under the effects of drugs, or the advanced stages of senile dementia, or in a coma, and so on. So, clearly, there are occasions when it is not possible to adhere to the principle of respect for autonomy. This is because some conditions are such that they disrupt a person's autonomy: they adversely affect a person's capacity for self-governance. A person with severe dementia in its later stages has had their capacity for self-governance so eroded by that disease that they may be unable to make decisions which they made routinely before becoming ill. The same can be said of severe mental health problems. A person in an acute attack of these may be incapable of self-governance and it is the task of those caring for such a person to try to restore that ability with the use of appropriate therapeutic strategies. A person with a severe learning disability may have only a very limited capacity for self-governance, depending upon the extent of the disability. With such a person, one should try to respect the autonomy of the person to an appropriate degree, but to work out what that is is plainly not easy and we will return to such problems in the next chapter. These remarks are simply aimed at reminding readers that it is not always possible to respect the autonomy of others.

Also, it is important to stress that there may well be occasions when it is justifiable to override the principle of respect for autonomy. Most obviously, the principle of respect for autonomy may be overridden when a person exercises autonomy in a way that will harm others (perhaps by assaulting them). The obligation to respect autonomy is not without limit, and there are, as just noted, situations in which it is justifiable to override the principle of respect for autonomy, even when a person is autonomous. Next, though, it is necessary to consider the concept of competence.

Competence

Thus far, little mention has been made of the concept of competence. It is also fair to say that texts on nursing ethics generally do not attempt to distinguish the concepts of autonomy and competence (Benjamin and Curtis, 1986; Melia, 1989; but see O'Brien and Golding, 2003). But how do these concepts differ, and why is the concept of competence important?

It was pointed out earlier that, 'autonomy' can be taken to mean 'self-governing'. But, clearly, from the fact that one is autonomous and thus self-governing, it does not follow that one is necessarily competent. Whilst 'autonomy' refers to a general capacity of an individual (that of self-governance), 'competence' refers to more specific abilities, such as those involved in the performance of specific tasks (Beauchamp and Childress, 2009, p. 112). For example, nursing students may be autonomous in the sense of being able to make their own way to work, to decide which clothes to wear, to decide how much money to take to work and so on. Yet, in spite of these facts, a student might not be competent to take a person's blood pressure. Similarly, the student, though autonomous, may not be competent to perform any number of tasks: heart transplant operations, a service on a car, to give a lecture in nuclear physics, and so on. So, it is clear that being autonomous is not a sufficient condition for being competent; but it does seem that it is a necessary condition.

The relevance of this distinction between autonomy and competence to nursing ethics is that in many moral problems arising from nursing practice, the question of the competence of the patient is absolutely crucial. For example, in the kind of case referred to in the *Open Mind* article mentioned earlier, and discussed in the other references given, it would be much easier to justify preventing a patient from leaving the ward if they are not able to make a competent decision to leave. Conversely, it is much more difficult to justify standing in the way of the patient's wish to leave the ward if their decision to leave is a competent one.

Another example of a moral issue in the nursing context which centrally concerns the concept of competence is the issue of informed consent. Clearly, to give one's informed consent to undergo a medical procedure one has to be mentally competent to make that decision, one has to be competent to perform the task of making the decision. So, it is evident that the concepts of autonomy and competence, though related, are distinct, and that each is closely bound up with moral issues in nursing.

In continuing the discussion of competence, it will prove useful to say a little about factors which may affect a person's ability to make a competent choice, and to consider just how one might attempt to determine whether an individual is or is not competent. Factors which affect competence can be divided, very roughly, according to their physical or psychological nature.

Physical factors

Obvious physical factors which can affect a patient's competence include drug intoxication and neuronal damage. A person who has consumed large amounts of drugs which affect the nervous system – for example alcohol or tranquillizers – may clearly have their capacity to reason impaired; as might a person who has sustained significant damage to their nervous system either due to physical trauma or disease. So such a person may not be competent to make a decision regarding their care.

It is important to bear in mind that a person has not lost the capacity to be autonomous until the parts of the nervous system necessary for rational thought are irreversibly destroyed (as is the case in humans in persistent vegetative states). Hence, individuals who are under the influence of drugs, or who suffer impairment of cognitive function due to transient neuronal damage, still possess the capacity to make autonomous choices. It is simply that at that time the person is not able to exercise that capacity due to the effects of the drugs or neuronal damage.

Psychological factors

With reference to psychological factors affecting competence, we can identify anxiety, coercion and lack of information. If a person is extremely anxious, his capacity to make competent decisions is likely to be impaired. The point can be illustrated with an example – a case meeting to discuss whether a patient is to be discharged from a psychiatric hospital. At the meeting are ten or twelve people: a consultant, medical students, nursing staff, nursing students, social workers, occupational therapists and so on. The consensus of the meeting is that the patient is not yet ready for discharge. The patient is then invited into the meeting, informed of the collective opinion and asked if he thinks it best that he stay in hospital a little longer. The patient says 'Yes'.

Can the patient's decision be regarded as a competent one? Many people find it difficult to speak in front of groups of other people – especially those composed of such powerful figures as consultants, nurses and social workers. It is possible that the patient will feel so anxious in the situation just described that his main objective will not be to answer the question after consideration of relevant information, but simply to escape from the stressful situation. Such an anxiety-provoking situation as that just described is, to say the least, not conducive to the patient making a competent decision. The example indicates how anxiety can adversely affect one's capacity to make competent decisions. Examples such as this indicate how important it is that nurses take their advocacy role seriously (NMC, 2008). One hopes that the nursing staff would ensure that the patient has expressed his real view, and point out to the other health care professionals the intimidating nature of the situation when it is seen from the patient's perspective.

It is also important to note that a person who 'chooses' one course of action as opposed to another due to coercion, cannot be said to have made a competent choice. Faulder (1985) points out that it is a feature of the logic of choosing that one has at least two courses of action open to one. The *Open Mind* article referred to earlier describes situations in which people who are in-patients in psychiatric hospitals may choose to discharge themselves. Upon voicing this choice, they are informed that if they try to do so they will be forcibly detained under the Mental Health Act (1983 as amended 2007). A person who consequently omits to pursue their intended course of action, cannot be said to have made a competent decision to stay on the ward. They will have been coerced into staying (Beauchamp and Childress, 2009, p. 133).

It was noted earlier that a clear distinction can be made between the notions of competence and autonomy. In explication of that distinction it was pointed out that a student nurse may be autonomous but not be competent, say, to take the blood pressure of a patient – the student may not know how to use a sphygmomanometer. In this example, the student is autonomous but lacks the practical and theoretical knowledge necessary to take a patient's blood pressure. Similarly, it was suggested that a student nurse may be autonomous but lack the competence to give a lecture on nuclear physics. In this case, the student lacks the knowledge to be able to give the lecture. Suppose this distinction is applied to examples relating to the taking of medication and the giving of informed consent. Given that it is evident that knowledge of specific information is necessary for a person to make a competent decision, it is plain that a person needs to know relevant information before he is in a position to make a competent decision to take or refuse medication. The expression 'relevant information', here, can be taken to include, minimally, the name of the drug being prescribed, the dosage, the benefits of taking the drug and also any possible harmful side effects. Just as the student nurse in our earlier example requires certain relevant information before being competent to take a patient's blood pressure, so patients require certain relevant information before they can make competent decisions to take medication prescribed for them.

Consider now the relationship between competence and the giving of informed consent. Again, possession of certain information is necessary for one to make a competent decision. So, a person is only in a position to give informed consent to undergo a particular medical procedure when in possession of relevant information. Plausibly, this includes information relating to the nature of the proposed medical procedure, its anticipated benefits and any attendant risks associated with the procedure. It is especially important to stress that a person who simply signs a consent form without reading it, and who is not in possession of the information just described, cannot be said to have given informed consent. They may have given their consent, but not their informed consent and it is the latter which is required from both legal and moral perspectives.

It may be added, here, that there seems to be a clear role for nursing staff in relation to the issue of informed consent. Nurses can perform an advocacy role by ensuring that people actually do give informed consent when they sign consent forms.

Determining competence

As seen earlier, it may be the case that a person lacks competence due to physical rather than purely psychological factors. For example, they may have senile dementia to such an extent that they are frequently – perhaps permanently – in a disoriented state. Thus, it may be the case that even if attempts are made to furnish the person with relevant information concerning a proposed treatment, their state may be such that he or she is unable to understand it, and that this is due to neuronal degeneration. Similarly, a person with a severe mental health problem may be so confused or deluded as to be judged incompetent to consent to (or refuse to undergo) a particular treatment.

Further, consider that one is a nurse working with elderly patients, some of whom are extremely confused. Suppose that one of them wishes to leave the ward, and it is feared that they will come to some harm as a consequence of their confused state. From the moral perspective, much hinges on the question of whether the decision of the patient is a competent one. If the decision is one which is competently made, it is much more difficult to justify trying to prevent them from leaving the ward (since autonomous persons are generally not prevented from undertaking potentially harmful acts, especially if they make competent decisions to engage in such acts). If the patient's decision is not competent, then it is much easier to justify preventing them from leaving the ward (see the next chapter for an extended discussion of such cases). Moral problems such as these make acute the need for criteria of competence.

One set of such criteria has been described by Beauchamp and Childress (2009). Strictly speaking, they propose criteria of incompetence: if a person fails the relevant 'test' – for example, being unable to make a choice, as in item 1 below – then the person is not competent to make the relevant decision. The criteria listed by Beauchamp and Childress are as follows:

1. Inability to express or communicate a preference or choice;

2. Inability to understand one's situation and its consequences;

3. Inability to understand relevant information;

4. Inability to give a reason;

5. Inability to give a rational reason (although some supporting reasons may be given);

6. Inability to give risk/benefit-related reasons (although some rational supporting reasons may be given);

7. Inability to reach a reasonable decision (as judged, for example, by a reasonable person standard). (Beauchamp and Childress, 2009, pp. 114–15; see also Buchanan and Brock, 1990.)

Note that these 'tests', are increasingly demanding; the criterion set out in item 6 is clearly more demanding than that set out in item 1. By item 6, a person counts as incompetent if he is unable to give reasons in support of and against (say) undertaking a particular course of action – perhaps discharging himself. But in item 1, a person only counts as incompetent if he is unable to indicate a preference. Thus, conceivably, a parrot could count as competent according to item 1, and not competent according to item 6 – provided the parrot could say 'yes' or 'no' when appropriately prompted.

Beauchamp and Childress state the criteria in the negative since they consider positive criteria of competence too problematic. However, in spite of their reservations, let us reconstrue their negative criteria positively:

1. Ability to express or communicate a preference or choice;

2. Ability to understand one's situation and its consequences;

3. Ability to understand relevant information;

4. Ability to give a reason;

5. Ability to give a rational reason;

6. Ability to give risk/benefit-related reasons;

7. Ability to reach a reasonable decision (as judged, e.g., by a reasonable person standard).
(With apologies to Beauchamp and Childress, 2009).

The character of the criteria still remains: test 1 is highly undemanding, whilst test 7 is much more demanding.

Test 1. Here, a person counts as competent if he or she is able to say 'yes' or 'no' (or shake or nod their head or communicate the choice in some other way, such as opening their mouth to receive food).

Test 2. In this case, a person is competent if he can understand his predicament and its consequences. Presumably, some visible evidence would be required to determine whether or not a person understood his situation. Of course the expression 'understand his predicament' or 'situation' is far from clear. One way in which it might plausibly be construed would be to imply knowledge of one's location – spatial and temporal. Even this requires further clarification, since if someone is asked their location and answers 'Earth', then they are correct!

More appropriate criteria might reasonably require knowledge of (a) the present address of the person, and (b) a rough idea of the time and year. With respect to (a), this need not require that the person whose competence is in question be able to give the exact postal address, say, of the hospital or community home at which they are staying. But it does seem reasonable to require that the person knows at least where they are, even if this is simply that they know they are in hospital. If they know the name of the town, and the name of the hospital or community home at which he or she is presently staying then this is stronger evidence of competence. With respect to (b) -temporal location – it seems unreasonable to require exact knowledge of this. At the time of writing this passage it is 12.55p.m., 13 June 2008, but it is a struggle to recall the exact date. Also, it is common for people to make mistakes concerning the exact year – one might easily claim that it is 2006 and forget that it is 2008. For these reasons, it seems that only an approximate knowledge of one's temporal location should be expected.
One might begin by asking the patient if he knew the approximate time of day, then continue by asking the day, month and year. It seems

excessively harsh to require exact knowledge of all these facts, but for it to be said that a person has a rough awareness of his temporal location one would expect that the person is not more than ten years out in answer to the question 'What year is it?', and is no more than five months out in answer to the question 'What month is it?' Whether or not the person needs to be asked which day of the week it is may plausibly depend upon other factors – say, whether the purpose of the trip out is relevant to the day of the week. If the person intends to use the Post Office and it is Sunday, there may be grounds to doubt that the person knows his temporal location.

In short, there is no simple means of determining whether a person knows his spatio-temporal location. But for it to be plausible that a person understands his situation, it can be expected that the person is able to offer a rough idea of his spatial location, and a rough idea of the year, month and time of day. These are minimal requirements to be met by a person said to understand his situation.

In Beauchamp and Childress's statement of criteria for determining competence, they employ the phrase 'understand one's situation and its consequences' (2009, p. 114). I have construed what it is to 'understand one's situation', perhaps, more broadly than they intend. Since, on the interpretation set out above, understanding one's situation amounts to knowledge of certain spatio-temporal facts, how should the second part of the expression be interpreted ('and its consequences')? If one was aware that one could not walk due to some severe health problem, yet one tried to walk, this might show lack of understanding of the consequences of one's situation, and so be taken to indicate incompetence as opposed to competence. So competence would involve understanding that one is, say, at risk of possible harm if one pursues a certain plan of action (e.g., going for a walk).

Test 3. This concerns the ability to understand relevant information. Beauchamp and Childress's discussion of competence arises in the wider context of a discussion of autonomy and informed consent. Hence, they point out that it is necessary that a person deemed capable of giving informed consent to undergo a medical procedure is able to understand information relating to that procedure. In the wider context, we may construe the test as relating to a client's capacity to understand information relating to, say, the risks of going for a lone walk (if the person suffers from confusion), or wishes not to take medication or wishes to discharge himself. For a person to make decisions of this nature competently, it is necessary that the person is able to understand information relevant to the decision (e.g., the risks and benefits of pursuing the desired course of action).

Test 4. The ability to give a reason requires that the person be able to support an expressed preference with a reason. Suppose a person is asked 'Would you like to come to the shops?' A person who simply answers 'Yes' or 'No' has not given a reason. To return to the parrot referred to in the discussion of test 1, a parrot may be trained to answer 'Yes' or 'No' to questions, without the presence of any understanding on the parrot's part. Hence, it is plausible to suppose it is necessary for a person to be able to offer a reason in support of undertaking a course of action, or undergoing some medical procedure. For example, suppose that a person upon being asked to sign a consent form to undergo ECT (electro-convulsive therapy) simply said 'Yes', and signed the form without reading it. That would not constitute evidence of the person's competence to sign. Again, suppose a person responds to the question described above ('Would you like to come to the shops?') with the answer 'Yes': test 4 requires that the person offers a reason. Perhaps he might answer 'Yes. I feel like some fresh air'.

Test 5. With respect to this test, a person is required to be able to 'give a rational reason' (2009, p. 115). This is more demanding than test 4 since it requires that the reason offered by the subject be a rational one. The difference being appealed to here can be exhibited thus: a person is asked why he or she does not wish to sign a consent form to undergo ECT. The reason offered is that the persons carrying out the procedure are Martians. This constitutes a reason and hence the person has met the criterion of test 4. But, of course, the person has not provided a rational reason in support of his utterance, and does not satisfy test 5. Alternatively, suppose a different person refuses to sign a consent form to undergo ECT. When asked to supply a reason, this person replies that not enough information has been provided concerning the nature of the treatment and its likelihood of success. Evidently, this is a rational reason for refusing to sign. In the second case, the reason offered is relevant to the refusal, but in the first case the reason offered seems to radically conflict with reality: the possibility that the team carrying out the ECT are Martians is so remote as to border on the absurd.

Test 6. This test is still more demanding and requires a subject to 'give risk/benefit-related reasons' for or against a particular decision or course of action. Let us reconsider the person in the last example who refused to sign a consent form to undergo ECT on the (rational) grounds of insufficient information to make a decision. Suppose the person is given the information and then considers the advantages (the benefits) of undergoing the treatment and then the disadvantages (the risks). Advantages might include the lack of toxicity of the treatment; disadvantages might include the discomfort usually experienced preceding and immediately after the treatment. Such a person qualifies as competent under the criterion of test 6.

Another example may involve a patient who suffers from periods of confusion. Suppose they are presently staying on a hospital ward for confused elderly people. The patient states her intention to visit a friend who lives nearby, but the nursing staff are concerned that the patient might become confused whilst off the ward and come to some harm. They express their worries to the patient. He replies that he is aware of such risks, but is also aware of the benefits of taking a trip outside the ward independently. The patient again meets the criterion set out in test 6.

Test 7. This final test is the most demanding, and requires that the person be able 'to reach a reasonable decision (as judged, for example, by a reasonable person standard)' (ibid.). This goes further than test 6 in that it requires the person to arrive at a decision which is regarded as that which a 'reasonable person' would make. Test 6 requires only that a person considers relevant risks and benefits, and offers no view on the nature of the eventual decision.

A difficulty, perhaps serious, with test 7 centres on the lack of clarity in the appeal to a 'reasonable person' standard of evaluation. Consider, again, the patient wondering whether to undergo ECT. Suppose they meet the criterion set out in test 6. It would seem that there are only three possible decisions that could be made: to refuse the treatment, to have the treatment, or to defer making a decision; and that any one of these would be reasonable. So in this example, it seems that test 7 is redundant. Provided the person considers the relevant risks and benefits – as required in test 6 – the person counts as competent.

What of our other patient, the person who suffers periods of confusion but wishes to leave the ward to visit a friend? Again it seems, once the risks and benefits have been considered – as required in test 6 – there are only three options: to proceed with the visit alone, to reconsider, or not to go. As before, all three of these seem reasonable options.

It seems, then, in the light of consideration of these examples, that it is the criterion set out in test 6 which is of greatest importance in determinations of the competence of clients. It needs to be noted that the criteria are wholly independent of age-related considerations. A person may be competent to decide against life-saving treatment at age 6, and not competent to do so at age 16 or 60. The application of this criterion is independent of the age of the person whose competence is being called into question.

One further point here: both Beauchamp and Childress (2009) and Buchanan and Brock (1990) suggest that criteria for determining competence should, to some extent, be decision-relative. That is to say, the criterion of competence the person is expected to satisfy is related to the seriousness of the decision being made. So, the less important the decision, the less demanding the criterion of competence required. And for important decisions correspondingly higher criteria of competence are required. For example, consider two situations. In the first, a person who is extremely confused is asked whether they would like a cup of tea or coffee. The person does not answer. The question is put differently: 'Would you like a cup of tea?' The person now answers 'Yes' (or for that matter, 'No'). The person meets the criterion of competence set out in test 1. Is there any point in trying to determine whether the person satisfies any of the more stringent criteria? Surely not – provided, of course, that nothing of importance hinges on the decision, for example that the tea contains arsenic or the person has a potentially fatal allergy to tea, and so on.

Consider now, though, cases in which people have more weighty decisions to make – such as in those examples recently discussed – decisions which could seriously affect an individual's safety or well-being. It seems entirely reasonable that more stringent criteria are required, so that the more important the decision, the more stringent the criterion of competence required. It is important to note, though, that as suggested above, the most demanding criterion is that of test 6. Considerations given above suggest that the criterion described in test 7 is redundant.

Considerable time has been spent, then, on the notions of autonomy and competence. The reason for this is that they are so crucial to what follows and in moral decision-making in nursing ethics that they require lengthy treatment. In fact, much more could be said in relation to either of these notions. However, let us now move on to consider a second level-three moral principle, that of beneficence.

The principle of beneficence

According to Beauchamp and Childress (2009, p. 197), the principle of beneficence 'refers to a statement of moral *obligation* to act for the benefit of others'.

(Strictly speaking they discuss two principles of beneficence, the one just described and a principle of 'utility' (2009, p. 197) by which they mean an obligation to weigh up harms and benefits and act in the way that leads to the most benefits. For present purposes we can ignore this and run together the two principles so that acting for the benefit of others includes acts which result from assessment of both harms and benefits. To illustrate, a young baby may be inoculated against mumps. This may produce some harms but overall benefits would be expected to outweigh any harms incurred in almost all cases. The principle of beneficence would be one kind of justification for such an act.)

The relevance of this moral principle to nursing ethics should be evident. It was seen in Chapter 1 that all nursing actions can be regarded as having a moral dimension: most of such actions are (or ought to be) for the ultimate benefit of patients and clients. The NMC Code (2008) states that nurses have a professional obligation to: 'protect and promote the health and wellbeing' of those in their care. It is reasonable to regard this as falling under the obligations of beneficence since when one's health and well-being are promoted, one is benefited.

With regard to the extent to which nurses are obliged to act in accordance with this principle, as the code makes plain it is required of them when they are on duty, and perhaps also when they are off duty. The previous NMC Code referred to a professional duty to 'provide care' in an emergency even when off duty (clause 8.5, 2004). This does not appear explicitly in the 2008 code, though it is stated that as a nurse you must 'uphold the reputation of your profession at all times' (NMC, 2008).

Further, the older UKCC Code (1992) used to make it plain that nurses are obliged to have regard to the workloads on their colleagues, and to ensure that these are not so extensive as to constitute 'an abuse of the individual' (UKCC, 1984; cf. clause 13, UKCC, 1992). It seemed, thus, that the obligations of beneficence to which nurses were then subject extended to the well-being of colleagues. This is slightly weakened in the NMC 2004 code which instead pointed to a highly general 'duty to colleagues'. (It looks to be weakened still further in the NMC Code 2008, though obligations to 'colleagues' still feature.) Given this, a question arises: how are we to understand the term 'colleagues'? Does this cover only those people in one's immediate working environment – say, the ward one works on, or one's colleagues in a community team? Or do the beneficent obligations extend to all the nurses in the hospital or Trust within which one is employed? Perhaps the term 'environment of care' (NMC, 2004) can help here. It may then be suggested that the nurse's obligations of beneficence extend only to those colleagues who work within the nurse's environment of care. This is certainly more realistic – though not entirely without ambiguity. How broad is the 'environment of care'? This question is also raised by the 2008 code since it refers to the importance of protecting the health and well-being not just of patients, but of 'the wider community' (NMC, 2008).

Related to the last point is this. Just as the extent of the nurse's obligations of beneficence to colleagues may be unclear, so too is its extent to patients. For example, is the nurse equally responsible for the well-being of the patient on neighbouring wards as for the well-being of patients on her own ward? It seems plain that the nurse is most responsible for the wellbeing of those clients on her own ward (equivalently, her case-load). But, equally, if a nurse is aware of, say, gross malpractice on a neighbouring ward, then the nurse's obligations of beneficence extend to the patients suffering due to that malpractice and she has an obligation to try to protect those patients (NMC, 2008). Plainly, ignoring ill-treatment of patients on a neighbouring ward would constitute a failure to 'uphold the reputation' of the nursing profession.

In short, it seems that the nurse's most weighty obligations of beneficence are to those patients and colleagues with whom she has closest professional practice and for whose well-being she is formally responsible (due to the NMC Code). But, given this, the nurse still has obligations of beneficence – less weighty than those just referred to – to colleagues and patients who may not fall within the nurse's immediate sphere of responsibility (indeed, as we have seen, these extend to 'the wider community' (NMC, 2008).

Two other points relating to the principle of beneficence are these. First, it is evident that other moral principles serve to constrain the obligations referred to by this principle. (I am indebted to Gillon [1985] for the following way of characterizing the relation between the principle of beneficence and other moral principles.)

For example, suppose a patient expresses an intention to continue to smoke in spite of his having chronic lung disease. Obligations of beneficence include obligations to promote well-being. This might reasonably be taken to involve attempting to prevent the patient from smoking – 'for his own good' as one might say. So obligations of beneficence appear to support preventing the patient from smoking – even if this is against his wishes. But obligations of beneficence clearly run up against, and conflict with, obligations to respect autonomy here. If the patient wishes to smoke, and if his decision is a competent one, then the obligations of respect for autonomy indicate that the patient's wishes should be respected. Here is a classical moral dilemma in nursing ethics (and health care ethics generally), which is caused by a clash between obligations stemming from different moral principles – in this case the principles of respect for autonomy and of beneficence. This particular type of clash will receive extended discussion in the next chapter, and so will not be discussed further here.

The second point concerning the principle of beneficence is this: actions which place obligations of beneficence above those to respect autonomy are describable as paternalistic actions. Roughly, they are actions for the good of someone else, but which conflict with that person's own wishes. In short, it can be said that the principle of beneficence serves to support paternalistic actions (a fuller discussion of this point follows in the next chapter).

We have not yet enlarged upon the issue of just what it is to benefit someone. The import of the term 'benefits' as it features in the principle of beneficence needs some comment. The benefits referred to can be understood, minimally, as physical and psychological benefits. Of course, it is unclear if these two types of benefits are, ultimately, separable. But it needs to be borne in mind that simply attending to physical problems can fall short of conferring benefits on patients. For example, it may be that the patient's physical problems have a psychological cause – liver damage may be due to alcohol poisoning and the consumption of alcohol due to depression. So it is important to construe 'benefits' quite broadly here. Also, it can be important to think of longer-term benefits too. A smoker might hold the view that the benefits of smoking are so great that they are worth the risk of the harms which, if he is lucky, he *might* escape. And he may even prefer a shorter 'pleasure filled' life to a longer one bereft of the pleasure he derives from smoking. So it can be very problematic to determine just what it is to try to 'promote the wellbeing' of patients. This is because the notion of well-being has a subjective aspect to it which can make it difficult to know what course of action best promotes the well-being of another person.

When this subjective aspect to well-being is noticed one can be led to the conclusion that obligations to promote well-being must always coincide with obligations to respect autonomy. This is because, it is argued, all one's choices express one's preferences and seek to secure one's best interests, since, after all, one is best placed to judge what lies in one's own best interests. The kind of example that the smoker described above provides may be pointed to in support of such a line of thought. In light of this kind of argument it may be proposed that the principle of beneficence is in fact a redundant principle because all the 'work' it does – all the moral terrain it covers – is covered by the principle of respect for autonomy.

There are at least two ways of responding to this seductive argument. The first is to point to situations where a patient lacks autonomy but there remains an obligation to act in the patient's best interests. So for example, a baby born very prematurely is obviously not able to express a view about what is in her best interests, but it remains possible to base any treatment decisions on the basis of consideration of her best interests. So this shows that the principle of beneficence is not redundant, at least in situations where a patient lacks autonomy.

The second response tackles the more difficult problem of showing how obligations of beneficence and autonomy need not coincide even though a patient is autonomous. I doubt that a compelling case can be made to show this, but nonetheless a convincing one can be. To see this, imagine that the line of argument described above is correct and that choices always reflect a person's own view about what is in their best interests. If this is the case it would be self-contradictory to say 'I did X even though I knew it was not in my best interests'. But this does not seem to be a statement which is self-contradictory. It may even be informative, for example, when someone is explaining why they acted in a particular way. Thus suppose a patient drinks well above the government recommended units of alcohol per week. She confides to a nurse that she knows she drinks too much and is trying to cut down on the amount she drinks. She confides further that she even had a drink last night. You ask her why and she says something like this 'I know it is not in my best interests to drink, but I just felt like one. I regret it now.' The statement is coherent because of the possibility of making decisions which one knows are not in one's best interests, even as one conceives of these oneself. If one's decisions always coincided with what one took to be in one's best interests, the patient's statement would be meaningless. It would involve the assertion of something that could not asserted (i.e., that one pursued a course of action that one knew not to promote one's best interests). Such a view could not be asserted because it would be self-contradictory. Yet most of us would be confident that the statement is not contradictory, and that the patient's expressions of regret, if sincere, are meaningful.

Now that this 'redundancy' argument can be set aside consider a case example which illustrates the problem in determining best interests. The example is that of a patient aged 60 who has been admitted with a heart problem which is now stabilized following a stay in the CCU. The patient feels well and is keen to go home. The health care team, though, want the patient to remain in hospital for further investigations as the cause of the heart problem remains unknown. They think it best for the patient to be referred for an angiogram. As there is a queue for this investigation, if the patient is to access it as soon as possible it is best for him to remain an in-patient, as the queue is shorter for these. If he goes home and is placed on a queue to have the investigation as an out-patient he might have to wait several weeks, perhaps 8 to 10. The patient is told that he has to remain in hospital as he needs to undergo further investigation. It is assumed that the patient will agree with the calculation made by the health care team to the effect that his interests are best promoted by remaining as an in-patient for at most three days so that the investigation can be carried out. So here obligations of beneficence, at least as far as the health care team are concerned, point so obviously to the 'in-patient' option, that the other option is not even mentioned to the patient.

What becomes clear later though, in the patient's care, is that had he been made aware that he could have had the investigation as an out-patient, even though there would have been a long wait for it, during which the heart problem might recur, he would have opted for the out-patient option. This is because, at least as far as the patient is concerned, being an in-patient in the hospital is such an unpleasant experience he would rather take the risks involved in the 'out-patient' option than remain in hospital any longer.

This case illustrates the difficulty in determining just what plan of care constitutes the most beneficent. For the patient, the benefits to his health that are likely to result from the in-patient option are not outweighed by the distress caused by the experience of being an in-patient (the lack of privacy, freedom, basic comforts, familiar surroundings etc.). The patient's own view is that the out-patient option is the most beneficent.

This kind of case points to the problem of determining how to act beneficently when the patient is competent. As the case has been described, the best option may have been for the team to explain the available options to the patient and listen to his opinion about which is best for him. But, the presumption was that the out-patient option is 'obviously' too risky and so there was no need to even mention that. This presumption clearly underestimates the distress that stays in hospital cause to some patients.

Assessments of beneficence are also needed, of course, when patients are not competent. Such a case was presented recently on the BBC programme 'Inside the ethics committee' (BBC, 28/8/07). It involved David, a man with very severe learning disabilities who had been diagnosed with cancer which was at a very advanced stage by the time of diagnosis. Treatment with chemotherapy would have been the usual treatment option offered to him were he capable of consenting to have it. The chances of his survival were less than 50:50. His learning difficulties were so severe that it was doubted he would co-operate with the treatment, which involved receiving regular doses of medication, for prolonged periods over three weeks. David's carers said he found any change in routine extremely distressing and that they were certain he would not tolerate the proposed treatment regime.

If one is caring for this person and seeks to act in his best interests, how can one try to assess what these are? An obvious route, asking the person themselves is closed as his learning disabilities are extremely profound. David cannot communicate in spoken or sign language, or by use of pictures and so on. Given this, the views of the people who know him best are the only source of insight into what is important to the person: How and to whom does he relate best?; What does he most enjoy?; What does he most dislike?; and so on. Such sources can help to construct a picture of what is in David's best interests. For if the interventions jeopardize these, then this would count against subjecting David to them especially when these harms are balanced against any probable benefits of the interventions.

In the end, the committee decided not to treat David and he died some five months later. The rationale seemed to be that having listened to the views of those who knew David best, it would be likely that the harms incurred by the treatment would be very great and would seriously damage those aspects of his life that made it worthwhile for him. So due to the inevitability of damaging David's relationship with his carers, and the significant risk that the treatment regime might not be effective anyway, it was decided not to treat him.

Of course, this decision is contestable. A counter-argument to it might run thus. Without the therapy David will certainly die. If he has it there is at least a chance for him to survive. If he does, then he can continue to enjoy those things that he enjoys now. So his interests are best promoted by his undergoing the therapy.

Evidently, those who knew David best did not think this to be a compelling case. As mentioned above, the prospects of success, plus the harms that undergoing the therapy would produce in David were thought to outweigh the considerations given in the counter-argument. This case is intended to illustrate how considerations relating to 'best interests' can proceed even when someone is not able to offer their own opinion about this. The case also illustrates the way in which benefits and harms can be weighed against each other.

Since the concept of harm has been introduced in this last example, let us now move on to the third principle, that of non-maleficence.

The principle of non-maleficence

This is defined by Beauchamp and Childress thus: 'The principle of nonmaleficence imposes an obligation not to inflict harm on others' (2009, p. 149). It is reasonable to claim that the principle underpins several of the major clauses in the NMC Code: '[you must] protect and promote the health and well being of those in your care' and '[you must] provide a high standard of practice and care at all times' (NMC, 2008). And to 'keep your skills and knowledge up to date' (ibid.). Obviously a central rationale for these clauses is to avoid harming patients by failing to practice competently, or by omitting to keep up to date with research that is relevant to clinical practice. Similarly, the code stresses the importance of acting quickly if you think a patient may be at risk (ibid.) and this similarly seems plausibly underpinned by obligations of non-maleficence. In minimizing risks to patients, one aims to reduce the extent of any harms they come to.

In their discussion of non-maleficence, Beauchamp and Childress construe harmful acts as those which 'set back the interests of the person affected' (2009, p. 152). So to illustrate this using the two examples discussed in the context of beneficence: Withholding the fact there was more than one treatment option available to the 60-year-old cardiac patient can be described as 'setting back' or thwarting (Beauchamp and Childress, 2001, p. 116) his interests in being in the environment he feels most comfortable in for as long as possible. Also, his interests are thwarted by not being given the full picture so that he is able to make a more informed response to his situation.

In David's case, those in support of denying him the chemotherapy may be said to have thwarted his interests – and thus harmed him – in terms of his longer-term survival. Or, in support of the decision, they may justly claim to be protecting his interests against the 'thwarting' of them that would occur should he be compelled to undergo the chemotherapy. Similarly, undergoing any significant physical or mental pain would count as a thwarting of one's interest in being pain free. So to harm people in these ways would be to fail to respect the principle of non-maleficence. Of course, if the benefits of undergoing the harms outweigh the harms incurred, then the transgression of non-maleficence may be justified.

It is important to highlight the difficulty of judging just what interventions might count as harming someone – 'thwarting' their interests. For most of us, given a choice between a life-saving blood transfusion and death, death would count as the greater harm; that would seem to thwart one's interests in the most drastic way possible. But a recent case in the United Kingdom highlights a difficulty that can arise when a person has a radically different conception of harm than is the norm. In October 2007 a young woman, Emma Gough, died shortly after giving birth to twins. Although the twins were born healthy, complications arose shortly after their birth and their mother needed a blood transfusion which, apparently, she refused due to religious reasons, she was a Jehovah's Witness. For her, apparently, receiving the blood transfusion would constitute a greater 'setting back' of her interests than would mortal death because receipt of the transfusion would entail her exclusion from the religion (BBC, 5/11/07 'Mother dies after refusing blood'). This tragic case illustrates that even an apparently simple moral rule 'don't harm others' can be extremely difficult to interpret and apply in practice because when it is applied, those applying it will typically be employing their own conception of harm. As this case shows, other people may work with conceptions of harm which differ radically from those we ourselves might employ.

More generally, it may be queried whether there is sufficient difference between the principles of non-maleficence and beneficence to warrant the employment of two distinct principles with accompanying distinct sets of obligations (cf. Beauchamp and Childress, 2009, p. 150). But the different import of these two principles can be exemplified by reference to the NMC Code (2008). For example, as noted above, the principle of beneficence refers to obligations to act in ways which promote the wellbeing of others. This principle can be said to provide the moral foundation of the clause '[you must]...promote the health and wellbeing of those in your care' (NMC, 2008). Suppose that instead of requiring nurses to promote the well-being of patients, the Code merely obliged nursing staff not to harm them. In other words, instead of obliging nurses to 'promote the health and wellbeing' of patients and clients', the code merely obliged nurses not to jeopardize the interests of patients and clients. Thus, patients entering hospital would not have their well-being promoted, but would merely not be harmed. Clearly, such a proposal seems absurd. Patients are referred to health care professionals to be made well, not simply to be protected from harm (though of course patients should expect this too). Obligations of beneficence seem much more demanding than those of non-maleficence. The latter merely oblige one not to harm others whilst the former oblige one to benefit others. So, obligations of beneficence would require us to help a needy, say homeless person, but obligations of non-maleficence would require us merely not to harm such a person. (See also Chapter 7 below on related issues.)

This account of the distinction between the obligations of non-maleficence and those of beneficence can help to clarify the import of phrases such as 'agreed standards [of care]'. Given acceptance of the point that obligations of beneficence are more pertinent to health care than are obligations of non-maleficence, it seems to follow that appropriate standards of care are those which foster the well-being of patients. Standards which merely provide a safe environment of care for patients can, thus, be shown not to constitute appropriate standards of care. Of course, the environment of care should be safe, and not harmful to patients, but as mentioned their main purpose in coming in to hospital or for seeking nursing care is to be benefited, not simply to 'not be harmed'. This is why stories regarding poor standards of hygiene in hospital wards are found so disturbing by people (see 'The ward smelt of diarrhoea', BBC, 11/10/07). They fear that there is more likelihood of them being harmed in hospital than of being benefited.

It has been noted here that the NMC Code asserts an obligation not to harm patients, yet routinely patients are subjected to harms. A person undergoing a physical operation such as an appendectomy sustains physical harm when the surgeon's scalpel cuts open their abdomen. Patients with mental health problems may be harmed by forcible admission to hospital or by taking toxic major tranquillizers. Of course there are numerous other examples of harms befalling patients as a planned consequence of regimes of health care; but clearly in many situations – especially in the case of, say, a competent person voluntarily agreeing to undergo an appendectomy – such transgressions seem easily justifiable. In the case of a competent person, the principle of non-maleficence may be justifiably overridden due to acceptance of the view that obligations to respect autonomy are weightier than those of non-maleficence. So obligations to act in ways requested by the person count for more than obligations not to harm them. Perhaps, even more obviously, the benefits of undergoing the appendectomy should outweigh the harms which may befall the patient if the operation is not performed.

More controversially, it may be claimed that obligations of non-maleficence can justifiably be overridden in order to protect a person from avoidable harms. Perhaps compulsory immunization programmes and compulsory detainment of persons under the Mental Health Act (1983) count as examples of such situations (we will consider cases such as these in detail later in Chapter 4). Still more controversially, it may be claimed that a person might justifiably be harmed in order to prevent harms befalling others. Compulsory immunization programmes seem to count here, as may the compulsory detention of people who have a dangerous, easily transmissible disease. Also, it could be said that it is justifiable to harm (by restraining) a violent patient in order to protect other patients and health care professionals. It is evident, then, that there are circumstances in which health care professionals may justifiably contravene their obligations of non-maleficence.

Acts and omissions

Thus far, the discussion of non-maleficence has focused on actions which involve intentional bodily movements the purpose of which is to bring about a specific, intended, state of affairs. The surgeon's action of cutting open a patient's skin to perform an appendicectomy clearly counts as an action of this kind. But it is possible to harm or wrong a person by virtue of what one omits to do – by omission – in contrast to harming a person by an intentional action – by commission. The NMC Code shows explicit appreciation of this point 'As a professional, you are personally accountable for actions and omissions in your practice...' (2008). Two examples of harming a person by omission are given below.

A person walking past a small, shallow pond notices a small child drowning in it. The child is well within reach and could be pulled out with minimal effort. In spite of the easy accessibility of the child and the fact that the person understands that the child's life is in danger, a conscious decision is made to walk past and do nothing to help the drowning child.

A second example involves a nurse who deliberately omits to provide an unconscious patient with medication without which the patient will die (insulin or digoxin perhaps). It is to be supposed that the patient is one for whom the nurse has clinical responsibility. The nurse simply omits to provide the prescribed drug in full knowledge of the consequences of such an omission.

Other examples include the following situations: allowing neonates to die by omitting to provide them with necessary nourishment (Kuhse and Singer, 1985); omitting to give a patient information necessary to make an informed decision regarding a treatment option; or omitting to prevent harms befalling patients due to mistreatment of them by other health care professionals. Also, perhaps, omitting to take action to prevent avoidable suffering to the patients who are in one's care.

So, it is clearly the case that we need to look a little further at the issue of harming others by omission as opposed to harming them by action (or 'commission' as it is sometime put). In fact, it has been asserted that there is a moral difference between harming another by omission and harming another by commission. The view that there is such a moral difference stems from the acts and omissions doctrine, the doctrine that

> [In] certain contexts, failure to perform an act, with certain foreseen bad consequences of that failure, is morally less bad than to perform a different act which has the identical foreseen bad consequences. (Glover, 1977, p. 92)

Thus, according to the doctrine, there is a morally significant difference between actively bringing about a state of affairs which harms another, and that state of affairs arising due to something one consciously omits to do. For example, suppose the prognosis of a very severely disabled baby is extremely poor – the baby is expected to survive for at most a month and during that time will experience great pain. Nurse A is in favour of bringing about the death of the baby by administering a lethal injection. Nurse B, the infant's parents, and the rest of the health care team favour simply omitting to provide the infant with nourishment necessary for its survival. According to the acts and omissions doctrine, the 'treatment' regime favoured by Nurse B and the others is morally less bad than the regime put forward by Nurse A – even though the different regimes have the same intended outcome.

Many nurses and doctors say they think withdrawing life-prolonging treatment is morally worse than withholding such treatment. Such a view seems supported by the acts and omissions doctrine. For if both options – withdrawing or withholding – lead to the death of the patient, according to the doctrine, it is 'less bad' that this consequence results from an omission (e.g., withholding of treatment) as opposed to an action (e.g., withdrawing of treatment).

However, the doctrine has been subjected to severe criticism (Wilkinson and Garrard, 2005; Beauchamp and Childress, 2009, p. 156). Critics argue that the factors which seem to make withdrawing treatment a moral wrong are present to an equal degree when life-prolonging measures are withheld. When treatments are withheld, they argue, there remains a direct causal chain between the decision to withhold and the death of the patient. So both of the factors which make withdrawing treatment wrong are present to an equal degree when treatments are withheld. This argument has led many to doubt the robustness of the doctrine. But abandonment of the acts and omissions doctrine might be thought to lead to some uncomfortable conclusions. For example, we tend to believe that there is a moral difference between, say, acting in such a way as to blind a person – say by poking his eyes out – and merely failing to prevent the onset of blindness even though this could have been prevented. Charities commonly remind us that a mere £500 donation can save a person's sight – typically a person in a poor country suffering from cataracts. Even though many who read this book could easily send such a donation, we omit to do so. Yet, we regard ourselves as morally distinct from a person who 'deliberately' causes the blindness of another person. If omissions are as morally reprehensible as commissions, there is no moral difference between ourselves and the person who 'deliberately' puts out the eyes of another. Perhaps fortunately, we do not need to possess a theoretical view on the acts and omissions doctrine – there are plausible arguments both in favour of it, and against it (Singer, 1993; Oderberg, 2000).

What is important to note for our purposes is that one can be morally responsible for actions one omits to perform, in addition to acts one does perform. The question of equivalence in degrees of moral responsibility is a difficult one and perhaps it would detain us too long to discuss this at length. Suffice it to say that even if, in one case, bringing about harms by omission is morally speaking as bad as bringing about such harms by commission, it does not follow that in all cases harms brought about by omission are as morally bad as harms brought

about by commission (indeed Glover's definition of it begins with the words 'in certain contexts' and hence, not necessarily in *all* contexts).

The principle of justice

This is the fourth and last of the level-three moral principles put forward by Beauchamp and Childress (2009). Their concern is with distributive justice; in particular, the distinction between distributions of health care that are just and those which are unjust. Reasonably enough health care itself can be regarded as a 'good' that is to be distributed – shared out – in some way. Most of us would think this should be done in a systematic manner, and not simply be a random distribution done without regard for fairness, or what people are entitled to, or what they have a right to and so on. By 'health care' it is meant, obviously, access to equipment, expertise, the time of health care professionals, access to drugs and so on.

The question 'What is a fair distribution of access to health care?' presupposes agreement about just what would count as a fair distribution; it presupposes a criterion of a fair distribution. To see this, consider that A and B are two people sharing a cake. A cuts the cake into four even quarters and then takes three of them, leaving only one left for B. B complains, 'that's not fair', and A responds by saying that as far as she is concerned it is a fair distribution of the cake. On the face of it this does seem an unjust distribution of the cake. The pair do not receive equal shares. However, we could elaborate the example by adding that A had not eaten at all that day and in fact had actually made the cake. So we might say the distribution is, after all, just. A deserves a larger share because she made the cake, and not only that, B has had plenty of cake that day whilst A has had none. What this indicates is that a distribution of a good can be just even though it is not one in which all affected receive the same amount of the relevant good. Also, the example illustrates that when thinking about justice, one is led to introduce concepts of fairness, and desert (what someone deserves). Let us consider each of these ideas of justice now.

Justice as desert

The suggestion here is that if, say, a person works hard and saves money for the purposes of enjoying retirement, it is just that the

person then does enjoy that retirement. The work that the person has put in and the sacrifices made, prompt us to judge that such a person deserves to have a happy retirement. It would be considered unjust, for example, if the pension scheme to which the person contributed became financially unstable and proved unable to provide the person with the pension due to him. Similarly, if a student nurse studies hard during his or her education and is enthusiastic on placement experiences, it may be judged that they deserve to pass their exams. So the thinking here seems to be that the efforts and time that one invests in something, entitles one to access to some 'good', whether this is health care, a nursing degree, a good pension, and so on. Of course, though, there is 'flip side' to thinking of justice in this way.

This is because we can apply the idea of desert negatively, so to speak, in that one might deserve to be punished having performed some terrible crime (this is justice in its 'retributive' sense). And further, in relation to health care, it may be said that a person 'deserves' not to be given scarce health care resources (transplant organs, for example) if the person has purposely pursued an unhealthy lifestyle. So it looks like interpreting justice wholly in terms of desert might lead to some fairly harsh conclusions (see also our discussion on resource allocation later (Chapter 4). So what about justice as 'fairness'?

Justice as fairness

Linguistically, as we were above, it seems obvious to articulate concerns involving justice in terms of fairness. Hence in the cake example we discussed, B's first appeal is that the distribution is unfair. But what is it to treat people fairly? It is commonly thought to require, at least, the equal treatment of equals. So, for example, suppose that a lecturer promises to give £5 to students who turn up for a particular lecture, but does not give all the students who turn up that amount of money. The students who are not given the money might complain they are not being treated fairly.

Stated a little more precisely, according to the idea of justice as fairness justice is done if equals are treated equally, and unequals treated unequally in proportion to relevant differences between them (this conception of justice derives from Aristotle, *Ethics*, and informs the discussion of justice by Beauchamp and Childress, 2009). So, in the case of the students who miss out on the £5, it may be claimed that all the students present at the lecture are equally entitled to the money since they are all present; hence 'equals' are receiving equal treatment. Students absent from the lecture, thus, would not receive the £5 since they are not 'equal', in the relevant sense, to the students present at the lecture. In this sense, equals are treated equally and unequals treated unequally and so the distribution of the £5 is a fair one.

A different example is the following: suppose a parent of twins allows one twin to stay up after 9.00 p.m. but the other is made to go to bed at that time. The second twin may claim to have been treated unfairly because 'equals' are not being treated 'equally' – that is, in the same way.

Relevant characteristics

What is going on in these examples is that some judgement is being made concerning what is to count as a relevant characteristic of the individuals involved, and a judgement made concerning the relationship of that characteristic to the action of the lecturer or the parent. In the lecturer example, since there is no relevant difference between the students present who receive the £5 windfall and those who do not, the latter group can claim to have been treated unjustly. Equivalently, the second twin may claim to have been dealt with unjustly due to there being no relevant difference between the twins.

But suppose we add some further details. In the lecturer case it may be conjectured that there is some difference between those students who do and those who do not receive the money. Perhaps the students who were given the money were particularly attentive and the lecturer wanted to reward them for this. If so, the action of the lecturer might now be regarded as just. This is because a relevant difference between those students who were given the money and those who were not has been identified. This difference is the justification appealed to in order to distinguish between the two sets of students: equals are being treated equally and unequals unequally. With respect to the twins example, it may be supposed here that the second twin had misbehaved in some way and that this comprised the distinguishing characteristic between the twins.

So, in relation to the characterization of justice as fairness offered above, evidently some judgement is required to be made concerning what is to count as a relevant characteristic in order that one is able to treat equals equally and unequals unequally. In our examples, it proved necessary to identify some criterion to justify treating one group of students differently from the other group, and to justify treating one twin differently from the other.

It is important to note that the actual formulation of the principle of justice (construed as an obligation to treat equals equally and unequals unequally) is silent as far as the vital question 'What *counts* as a relevant characteristic?' is concerned. All the principle obliges us to do is to treat equals equally (etc.), regardless of how it is determined which properties of individuals are relevant to judging them as equals. Hence, treating equals equally and unequals unequally requires some determination of the respect in which two individuals are equal or otherwise. They may both be equal in the sense that they are humans, or that they are male, or that they are Brazilian, or over 5 feet tall, or that they turned up for a lecture, and so on.

These rough and intuitive reflections on an ordinary understanding of the notion of justice prompt consideration of just which properties of individuals are to be taken into account in our evaluations of the fairness of particular actions (or policies, or laws). Some characteristics of individuals seem clearly not to be relevant in our moral judgements relating to justice. For example, suppose the lecturer claimed that the money had been distributed fairly. And, when asked what the basis for distinguishing between the two groups of students had been, he replies that it was the height of the students which constituted the relevant characteristic: all and only those students over 5 feet 10 inches were given the money.

From the moral perspective, one wants to ask what possible relationship there could be between one's height and one's entitlement to the £5. Imagine that such a proposal was advanced in relation to the question of how to distribute health care resources fairly. Suppose it is asserted that only those over 5'10' are entitled to receive such resources. Plainly, it would be absurd to judge that the height of the recipients was a central characteristic to be taken into account in the determination of a person's entitlement to health care resources. (This would be a form of 'heightism'.) Equally ridiculous characteristics could be put forward (and rejected); suppose it is proposed that health care resources are allocated only to those who are left-handed. Again, one would say that distributing resources on the basis of such a criterion would be wholly arbitrary from the moral perspective. Of course, there may be some special circumstances in which the height or left-handedness of a person may be relevant. For example in allocations of treatment involving human growth hormone (HGH) the height of the recipient is likely to be relevant. But the restriction of access to health care per se on the basis of height plainly seems absurd. What matters most, we might argue, is their clinical need, not their height. The HGH example just given is one in which height is related to clinical need.

Hopefully, the reader can discern where these points are leading to. In judgements relating to the just distribution of health care resources (or £5 notes, or privileges such as being allowed to stay up after 9.00 p.m.), certain characteristics of potential recipients of such resources are relevant, and other characteristics are not. So far, it has been suggested that (exceptional circumstances aside) height and 'left-handedness' cannot plausibly be regarded as relevant characteristics. For unless they can be shown to be connected to something that is relevant, such as clinical need, entitlement to health care resources should not be based exclusively on irrelevant characteristics such as the height of the recipient.

What of a policy that distinguishes between an individual's entitlement to health care resources on the basis of characteristics such as age, gender or nationality? Unless some kind of argument could be given to show that these characteristics of individuals are ones which legitimately affect their entitlement to health care resources, distinguishing between them on the basis of age, gender or nationality amounts to discriminating unfairly on the basis of characteristics which are not relevant from the moral perspective. Such a policy may be open, variously, to charges of ageism, sexism or racism.

It is evident from our reflections so far that a necessary feature of justice is impartiality. This is because, from the moral perspective, whether or not a person is a friend or relative of yours is not obviously a relevant moral characteristic of them. What matters are relevant characteristics such as what they have done, or what level of clinical need they have. The person making a just judgement, or who acts justly, is required not to favour individuals on the basis of considerations such as personal preference, or personal taste (see Singer, 1993, chapter 2, for more on this issue).

Impartiality and the NMC Code (2008)

An example from the nursing context may help here. The NMC states that

You must not discriminate in any way against those in your care.

And,

> You must treat your colleagues fairly and without discrimination. (2008)

The previous 2004 code stated

> You are personally accountable for ensuring that you promote and protect the interests and dignity of patients and clients, irrespective of gender, age, race, ability, sexuality, economic status, lifestyle, culture and religious or political beliefs. (2004)

In the terms with which we have been thinking about justice, the wrong that occurs when someone is discriminated against is this. They are denied something on the basis of characteristics which are not morally relevant. Thus to deny people access to dental care because they are women is plainly to deny them access to a good on grounds that are not morally relevant. It is akin to denying people access to dental care because they are left-handed. What is relevant is their clinical need for dental care. Which hand they use most frequently, or which gender they are is entirely irrelevant. So, the code is stressing the importance of distributing care in ways which are not discriminatory, that is, are based upon relevant characteristics of patients, not morally irrelevant ones.

Suppose it is claimed that nurses have stronger obligations to care for patients who are ill through no fault of their own, than to patients who are largely responsible for their own ill health, their illnesses are 'self-caused' let us say. Such a claim would involve the assertion that a defensible distinction can be made between the two groups of patients – those who bear no responsibility for the onset of their ill health and those who do.

Nurses have professional and moral obligations to all patients. According to the principle of justice nurses are obliged to treat equals equally and unequals unequally. This is implicit in the passages from the codes (2004, 2008) quoted above. The clauses require nursing staff to care equally well for patients regardless of their religious beliefs, gender, age, and so on. So the position stated in the code is that insofar as an individual is a patient, then nursing staff have obligations to treat that individual fairly. This entails not treating one patient any more or less favourably than another. The claim mentioned above, to the effect that individuals whose illnesses are self-caused are owed less by nurses, in terms of their obligations to care for them, can thus be seen to involve a violation of the NMC Code. By that clause, even if a patient's illness is self-caused this does not affect their entitlement to proper care by nursing staff.

With regard to the point made earlier relating to characteristics of individuals which are relevant from the moral perspective and those which are not, the following points may be made. It is evident that certain characteristics of people are ones which they have acquired by choice. At least they are characteristics to which a person voluntarily acquiesces Such properties might include being a supporter of Manchester United, being a footballer, being a father, being married, being a Conservative voter and so on. However, other characteristics of persons are not ones which they acquire with any degree of voluntariness. Examples here include, being human, being male (or female), being mortal, having white skin (or skin of any other colour), having brown eyes, being a certain age, being born at a particular time, being born at a particular location (town, country or continent), and possession of any other characteristic acquired non-voluntarily.

In assessing which characteristics of persons are most relevant from the moral perspective, it seems highly plausible to exclude those which the individual cannot help but possess – being a certain, age, sex or nationality for example. Given acceptance of this view, a general position close to that apparently advocated in the NMC Code seems to follow (NMC, 2004, 2008). When applied to the issue of how to distribute health care resources justly, the view implies that resources should be distributed without regard for such characteristics of individual patients. Hence, one's entitlement to a specific type of resource would be unaffected by one's age, sex and nationality (unless of course there is a connection between that characteristic and clinical need). The plausibility of such a position is one we will consider at greater length in Chapter 4.

The proposal just advanced seems supported by the earlier point that autonomy is a necessary condition of morality. That claim seems to support a view in which it is held that characteristics of people acquired non-autonomously (characteristics not acquired as a result of an autonomous decision) should not count as morally relevant in themselves (that is, as grounds for benefiting or burdening an individual).

In recent times, two rival theories of justice have received much attention; these are the theories put forward by Rawls (1971) and by Nozick (1974). To complete the discussion of the principle of justice, a brief outline of these two theories will now be provided and this will be followed in Chapter 4 by a consideration of the implications of the theories for the distribution of health care resources.

Rawls's theory

Rawls's theory identifies justice with fairness, and is generally characterized as an egalitarian theory. This is due to the fact that it seeks to distribute benefits and burdens equally among the members of a particular group – most obviously, among the members of societies. Rawls writes 'All social values...are to be distributed equally...' (Rawls, 1971, p. 62). It is also characterized as a contractarian theory (by Brown, 1986) – indeed, Rawls states that his theory owes much to the social contract theories put forward by Locke, Rousseau and Kant (Rawls, 1971, p. 11).

Clearly, if one seeks to identify justice with fairness one will need to clarify an understanding of the concept of fairness. By way of explicating this, Rawls describes a hypothetical 'original position' (1971, p. 17) in which individuals are able to characterize their view of what would constitute a just or fair set of social arrangements. Further, in making such a characterization, these individuals do so behind a 'veil of ignorance', which is to say that they do not know in advance what their position in such a set of arrangements will be. They will not know whether they are rich, poor, male, female, able-bodied, physically or intellectually impaired, intelligent or otherwise, and so on.

Rawls suggests two principles which would be deemed fair: (a) '[A] principle of greatest equal liberty' (1971, p. 124) according to which 'each person is to have an equal right to the most extensive basic liberty compatible with a similar liberty for others' (1971, p. 60); and (b) 'The principle of (fair) equality of opportunity' (1971, p. 124), according to which 'positions and offices [are] open to all' (1971, p. 60). Within (b) is included 'The difference principle', according to which, 'social and economic inequalities are to be arranged so that they are...reasonably expected to be to everyone's advantage' (1971, p. 60).

With respect to the first principle, this is evidently a fairly straightforward endorsement of the principle of respect for autonomy. The principle asserts that the only restrictions on the exercise of one's autonomy stem from infringements of the autonomy of others (see also Mill, 1863, p. 135). Not implausibly, Rawls supposes that such a principle will be chosen by subjects in the original position since they will choose not to have their own autonomy impinged upon by others.

As can be seen, the second principle divides into two parts. The first asserts equality of opportunity: positions in society will be open to any suitably equipped member of that society, and opportunities to acquire the appropriate equipment or qualifications will, again, be open to all. Evidently, then, social class, age, sex, and so on would not prove obstacles to candidacy for positions in society.

As for the second part of the (second) principle, inequalities in wealth and material possessions are permissible, but only insofar as the inequalities benefit the least well-off. Hence, such inequalities are legitimate only if the least wealthy are better-off in the presence of such inequalities than they would be in their absence.

As noted above, Rawls supposes that his principles will be acceptable to the subjects in the original position, behind the veil of ignorance. On the face of it, the supposition seems highly plausible. Given that the subjects do not know whether they will be rich, poor, healthy, sick, disabled, and so on, he supposes that they will opt for the set of arrangements in which their well-being will be protected in the worst set of circumstances (e.g., if they have a severe disability which prevents them from obtaining employment).

In the next chapter, some of the ramifications of the adoption of a Rawlsian criterion of justice for the allocation of health care resources will be discussed; for now, the second of the theories mentioned above will be considered, that proposed by Nozick (1974).

Nozick's theory

As seen above, the starting point of Rawls's theory is a position in which no participant has any possessions or a clear idea of their natural abilities. In contrast to this, Nozick's theory begins from a point in which it is recognized that subjects do have possessions – described by Nozick as 'holdings' (1974, p. 150) – and natural abilities, and it is from such a starting point that he develops his theory.

Nozick proposes that 'the subject of justice in holdings consists of three major topics'. These are matters relating to (a) ' the original acquisition of holdings', (b) ' the transfer of holdings', and (c) ' the rectification of injustice in holdings' (1974, p. 152). Hence, it is envisaged that there will be a principle of just acquisition of holdings, and a principle of just transfer of holdings. The third element serves to correct any transgressions of these principles of just acquisition and just transfer, which arise, say, by theft.

One of the merits of the theory noted by Nozick is that it is 'historical', which is to say that it takes into account how individuals come to possess their holdings. A person's holdings may have been inherited, or earned or justly acquired in some other way. Holdings are justly acquired if and only if they are acquired in a manner which does not contravene the principles of just acquisition or just transfer. This aspect of Nozick's theory accords with our intuitions regarding justice as 'desert' – at least in some ways; *pace* the application of the theory to inherited holdings (though, as noted, inherited holdings would be covered by the principle relating to the just transfer of them).

Nozick points out (1974, pp. 153–4) that other theories of justice seem not to take account of historical considerations in the way that his does. For example, a Utilitarian distribution of holdings would seem to consider at any one time the most equitable distribution of holdings at that time, as it accords, or fails to accord, with the principle of utility – regardless of events or patterns of distribution prior to that time. The justice or injustice of the distribution at a specific time would be wholly independent of historical considerations.

Similarly, egalitarian theories (such as that proposed by Rawls), when considered from Nozick's perspective, may be charged with ignoring relevant historical factors. For example as noted earlier, Rawls's theory asserts a 'difference principle' according to which any inequalities in holdings between members of a society are justified only if they benefit the least well-off. Thus, Rawls's theory places the 'end result', so to speak, of just distribution of holdings across a society above an individual's own historical claims to retain possession of those holdings. Thus, in Rawls's view, justice demands that holdings acquired, for example, by hard-working members of a society could justifiably be redistributed to less well-off members (as in taxation). Such a redistribution would only be legitimate in Nozick's account, if it had the consent of those with the holdings in the first place. Hence, if the principle of justice as applied in that society is construed in Nozick's terms, taxes due to be distributed to the least well-off can only be allocated to that group with the consent of individual, wealthy members of the society. In fact, Nozick writes, 'Taxation of earnings from labour is on a par with forced labour' (1974, p. 169). Also, with reference to the expression 'end result' as used above, it should be said that Nozick contrasts 'end-result' principles of justice with his own 'historical' principles (1974, p. 155).

So far, then, a brief description has been given of the main components of Nozick's theory, a motivation for it, and a consequence of its adoption. Those not persuaded of the merits of his theory are issued with a challenge by Nozick. Critics are invited to apply their own favoured theory of just distribution of holdings to an example supplied by Nozick; call this favoured schema of just distribution, Dl. (D1 may be a distribution in accord with Rawlsian criteria, or according to Utilitarian criteria, for example.) When this is done, he supposes, the theory of justice which most accords with the reader's intuitions concerning justice will be Nozick's own. The example is referred to as the 'Wilt Chamberlain' argument.

Nozick's Wilt Chamberlain argument

Nozick invites us to suppose that Wilt Chamberlain is a great basketball player (which he once was) and that when he plays home games, attendances are above average. Further, suppose that Chamberlain's crowd-pulling capacities are recognized and that he negotiates a contract in which 'twenty-five cents from the price of admission goes to him' (1974, p. 161). Nozick continues: 'Let us suppose that in one season one million persons attend his home games, and Wilt Chamberlain ends up with $250,000, a much larger sum than the average income and larger even than anyone else has. Is he entitled to this income? Is this...distribution [of holdings] unjust?' Call the resulting pattern of distribution D2 – that in which Wilt Chamberlain receives the large sum – and note that this results from our favoured pattern of distribution, D1. Also, bear in mind, of course, the fact that those who attend the games do so voluntarily, and autonomously choose to give their 25 cents to Wilt Chamberlain having previously been made aware of the details of his contract. Nozick's conclusion is that Wilt Chamberlain is entitled to the sum of money accrued, and that it is a just distribution of holdings. Further, it seems to be a distribution which accords with our intuitions concerning acquisition and transfer. The money acquired by Chamberlain is voluntarily given to him by parties concerned and so, it seems, must accord with any principles relating to the just transfer of holdings. Since D2 results from D1, and D2 is regarded as just, then D2 must also be a just distribution. (Nozick writes 'If D1 was a just distribution, and people voluntarily moved from it to D2...isn't D2 also just?')

However, a quite serious objection may be levelled at Nozick's theory, and this centres on the intuitions appealed to in the Wilt Chamberlain example. For example, suppose that Chamberlain earns £20,000,000 through the money-making scheme described above. Suppose, further, that a person who has such severe disabilities that they are unable to work and with no earning power is, as Kymlicka puts it, 'on the verge of starvation' (Kymlicka, 1990, p. 100). In Nozick's theory, there is no obligation on the part of wealthy citizens to aid the poor – even starving – citizens. Kymlicka suggests: 'Surely our intuitions...tell us that we can tax Chamberlain's income to prevent that starvation'. In Nozick's theory, those in possession of holdings can dispose of them in any way they choose, even if this results in the kind of situation just described. Hence, the point here is that Nozick's theory has an implication which conflicts so greatly with intuitions concerning justice that it is implausible to accept it. Also, it may be said that those who share the intuition appealed to by Kymlicka may take it to lend support to Rawls's theory. This is due to the role of the Difference Principle according to which, it may be recalled, great inequalities in material wealth are permissible only if the less well-off are better-off in their presence.

What can be taken from this brief outline of the two theories of justice is that two fundamentally different views regarding what constitutes justice can be well-supported. Further, when the two theories are applied to questions of resource allocation, they throw up different approaches. A Rawlsian view, for example, seems congenial to a schema of resource allocation which considers the health of all citizens. For, in Rawls's hypothetical original position the participants will be ignorant of their own health status and may be presumed to take this into account in their views concerning allocations of health care resources.

Thus, the Rawlsian view can be contrasted with Nozick's line. Nozick's theory seems more congenial to a schema of distribution of health care resources in which it is up to individuals themselves to arrange their own health care needs (presumably by insurance). Applied to health care, a Rawlsian approach, it seems, would be more likely to ensure the presence of mechanisms available to maintain the health of all the members of the state, and, hence, to ensure that the institutional structures necessary to implement that aim are in place (community care structures, hospitals, dental care, eye care, health information and promotion, and so on). This is because, it would be reasonable to suppose those in the original position, knowing they could fall ill at any time, would agree to have some kind of system for maintenance of health in the state. By contrast, a Nozickian approach to health care provision would very much leave it to the individual to arrange for their own health care needs to be met. Market forces would compete to provide the structures necessary to meet those needs. It seems most likely that nurses and other groups of health care professionals would be more favourably disposed towards a Rawlsian line rather than a position close to that put forward by Nozick. This is because in the Rawlsian position it seems more likely that the state apparatus necessary to implement health care would be in place; and, one imagines, this would appeal to those citizens who have an interest in and who care about the well-being of all the members of a state.

This completes our review of the four principles. What is to be done next is to try to argue that the principle of respect for autonomy is the most important of the four.

Respect for autonomy as the weightiest principle?

Having looked at each of the four principles in some depth, we return now to consider the argument that it is the obligations referred to by the principle of respect for autonomy that are the most important (or 'weighty'). This general position seems supported by the discussion of autonomy at the beginning of this chapter. There, it was claimed that the importance of autonomy can be derived from a number of considerations: (a) that many – perhaps most – people find paternalism objectionable; (b) that autonomy is highly valued and its absence considered psychologically unhealthy; (c) that autonomy seems a necessary condition of morality; (d) that the most serious crimes (murder, rape, theft) seem so because they involve profound violations of autonomy; this is mirrored by the fact that the most severe punishments involve similar violations; (e) that the point of health care, it seems, is to restore and foster autonomy. Further, (f) as seen, the legal position in the United Kingdom (and elsewhere) appears to reflect the weight accorded here to the principle of respect for autonomy. This is evidenced by the fact that autonomous persons are legally able to refuse even life-saving treatments, and that the consent of competent clients is legally required before treatment is permissible (except emergency treatment, of course, where the wishes of the client are not known). Finally (g), the emphasis given in the NMC Code (2008) to respecting the individuality of patients, to obtaining their consent, and respecting their confidentiality also points to the prominent place given to obligations to respect autonomy in that code (and previous versions). These points indicate that the principle of respect for autonomy is 'weightier' than the principles of beneficence or non-maleficence since competent decisions to refuse to submit to beneficent or non-maleficent actions are generally respected.

With regard to the principle of justice, as seen above, both of the theories considered retained a central place for respect for autonomy. More so, obviously in Nozick's account than in that developed by Rawls. But the significant point for present purposes is that respect for autonomy is the pre-eminent principle in each approach. Justice in these theories functions as a constraint on autonomy, as for example when the exercise of autonomy involves violations of the autonomous wishes of others. Also, justice is invoked when it is not possible to respect autonomy; for example, as may be the case in matters of resource allocation, justice is invoked solely because it is not possible to respect the autonomous wishes of those who require access to resources. These points also suggest that respect for autonomy is weightier than those of justice.

In support of this view, suppose, for the sake of argument, that justice is taken to be the most weighty of the four principles. We have seen that two of the most developed and well-known theories of this have respect for autonomy at their centre. So a position in which respect for autonomy is the most weighty moral principle would still be retained even if these approaches were adopted. Even though in Rawls version, as we saw, there are more limits to respect for autonomy than there are in Nozick's version. Suppose then a different conception of justice is taken, such as a utilitarian approach. In this autonomy can be transgressed in the most radical ways provided utility is maximized. As we saw above, an institution such as slavery could be justified on utilitarian grounds. Slavery of course constitutes one of the most serious assaults on autonomy conceivable. The fact that the wrongness of slavery seems so evident in fact highlights again the strength of adherence to respect for autonomy. So, these considerations lend support to the view that respect for autonomy is the weightiest of the principles (see also Gillon, 2003 who advances a similar case).

Although the strongest case available (as far as I can see anyway) has been put forward in support of the view just described, it is important to stress the limitations of it. There are no 'proofs' in ethics, so the line just developed cannot be claimed to be a truth in the way that we can show the truth of empirical facts such as water consists of H_2O or that it boils at 100 degrees C, or that humans have hearts etc. The most we can aim for are grades of plausibility and the line developed above seems plausible for the reasons given. But there are limitations of the 'autonomy-weighted' interpretation of the principle-based approach and it is important to highlight these now.

Consider again the arguments listed above as (a) to (g). All (except perhaps (c)) try to draw an ethical conclusion (that one ought to respect the autonomy of others) from empirical observations. Those exploited appeal to the law (d) (f), the NMC Code (g), some psychological observations (a) (b). These do not provide an absolutely compelling case in support of an autonomy-weighted view. To illustrate this, consider (a) again. A critic can perfectly reasonably claim that *nothing* follows from the fact that most of us find paternalism objectionable (even if it is true). It may be that we find paternalism objectionable, and we are mistaken to find it so. Or, that even though we happen to find it objectionable, nonetheless, it is morally the most defensible position.

It is also important to be reminded that one cannot respect the autonomy of newly born babies and of patients whose autonomy is compromised for various reasons. So there are further limits to the extent to which an autonomy-weighted approach can help in moral decision-making. Nonetheless in these types of cases, it is considered important to listen to the views of parents as far as the care of their children is concerned and this indicates a role for respect for autonomy in such circumstances. And, as the recent Mental Capacity Act (2005) now allows, even when one loses one's ability to make competent decisions, one can express views about the nature of the care one would want to receive or refuse by completing an advance decision before one becomes incompetent. So again, the importance of respecting autonomy is apparent even in these kinds of circumstances.

So, the limitations of the position advanced have been signalled. In spite of these, it remains the most plausible view in my opinion. I am persuaded by Beauchamp and Childress that a credible approach to morality must start from and be constrained by 'ordinary morality'. Also, the idea that respect for autonomy should generally be subordinated to obligations of beneficence and non-maleficence is not persuasive for the reasons given above (which again refer to existing moral practices and attitudes and so have limited force).

Hence, the position outlined in this chapter can, for obvious reasons, be described as an 'autonomy-weighted' principle-based approach. Some further criticisms of the approach are discussed in Chapter 5. For now, the chapter closes with a discussion of the close links between the NMC Code and the kinds of obligations referred to by the four principles.

The principles and the NMC Code (2008)

The code gives the 'Standards of conduct, performance and ethics for nurses and midwives' (NMC, 2008); and, it replaces the previous 2004 code. As it is presented, the new code highlights four key clauses. Each clause forms the heading of a page and is followed by several sub-clauses. All clauses are preceded by the statement 'The people in your care must be able to trust you with their health and wellbeing. To justify that trust you must...'

- make the care of people your first concern, treating them as individuals and respecting their dignity;

- work with others to protect and promote the health and wellbeing of those in your care, their families and carers, and the wider community;

- provide a high standard of practice and care at all times;

- be open and honest, act with integrity and uphold the reputation of your profession.

There are four other clauses which appear on the opening page of the code, but are not highlighted with bullet-points, the first two of these are as follows:

As a professional you are personally accountable for actions and omissions in your practice and you must always be able to justify your decisions.

You must always act lawfully whether those laws relate to your professional practice or personal life.

The other two clauses remind the nurse that failure to comply with the code may jeopardize the nurse's registration, and lastly there is a reference to further guidance at the NMC website.

As seen the clauses in the NMC Code of Professional Conduct (NMC, 2008) attempt to set out the 'standards for conduct, performance and ethics' (ibid.). It was pointed out in Chapter 1 that all nursing acts have some ethical dimension to them, since all such acts have moral goals: they aim at helping others, relieving their pain, promoting their well-being and so on.

We will now highlight the close connections between the clauses in the NMC Code and the principles and rules discussed so far. To do this, let us consider the four main, bullet-pointed clauses in turn, together with a selection of their sub-clauses. The first main clause is: 'The people in your care must be able to trust you with their health and wellbeing. To justify that trust you must...make the care of people your first concern, treating them as individuals and respecting their dignity'.

One can see the principle of respect for autonomy providing a moral basis for key aspects of this clause. To treat a person as an individual will involve at least the kinds of obligations captured in the principle of respect for autonomy. Thus it will be important to listen to patients' views about their condition and their care, and also, of course, to provide them with information so that they are able to make decisions about treatment options. Obligations to respect confidentiality and to gain patient's consent are also stressed under this main clause. Again it can be pointed out that the importance of these derives from the importance of respecting autonomy. Thus a key aspect of respecting confidentiality is to ensure patients still have some control over where sensitive information about them goes. The obligation to keep such information confidential thus is part of respecting the autonomy of patients. A similar story can be told about the relationship between the obligation to obtain the consent of patients and respecting their autonomy. Seeking of consent acknowledges that it is the patient who has control over who has access to their body.

The second main clause states that, as a nurse or midwife you must 'work with others to protect and promote the health and well-being of those in your care, their families and carers and the wider community'. The references in this to protection and promotion of health and well-being plainly can be understood in terms of the principles of non-maleficence and beneficence. To protect the health and well-being of another is to ensure they are not harmed. And to promote their health and well-being is to try to benefit them. There are other sub-clauses under this heading which point to the importance of other concepts which are directly related to the four principles, for example, 'best interests', the obligation to 'treat your colleagues fairly and without discrimination' and the importance of maintaining 'the safety of those in your care' (ibid.).

The third main clause indicates nurses and midwives must 'provide a high standard of practice and care at all times'. And again it seems reasonable to suggest this can be explicated in terms of the four principles. Thus a high standard of care respects the autonomy of patient, promotes their well-being, prevents them from harm and treats them fairly. Protection of confidential information is also mentioned again here.

According to the fourth main clause, a nurse or a midwife must 'be open and honest, act with integrity and uphold the reputation of your profession'. The main principles which underpin the clauses in this part of the code include respect for autonomy and justice. Thus to be honest includes respecting the autonomy of other, being truthful with them. Justice involves being fair in one's dealings with others, colleagues, patients and their relatives.

Some clauses in the code make reference to concepts which seem difficult to explicate in terms of the four principles, for example those referring to ideas such as trust and dignity. Having said this, I think it is still possible to interpret even these clauses in terms of the principles. With regard to trust, this is very closely tied to truth-telling, and obligations to be truthful as set out in the veracity rule, stem from obligations to respect autonomy. In general in relation to trust, obligations of fidelity, would be those that would 'mop up' any obligations not encompassed within those of respect for autonomy. These remaining moral considerations would include obligations relating to prevention of harm and of benefiting patients.

With regard to dignity, this is less easy to deal with as can be illustrated now. This is because to respect a person's dignity seems to amount to more than simply not harming them. To see this, suppose that a patient is unconscious, or perhaps even in a state of permanent unconsciousness (e.g., a persistent vegetative state). Suppose further that nursing staff are washing the body of the patient, and that this is done without drawing screens around the patient, so that other patients can see what is occurring. When the nurses have finished washing the patient they cover him up again.

In this example the patient is not harmed, the procedure causes no pain or discomfort. The procedure may even be beneficial to the patient in terms of its preventing tissue break down and in keeping him clean. Yet, to expose the patient's naked body for all to see without any attempt to protect the patient's body from the gaze of others (patients, their relatives, hospital staff unconnected with the patient being cared for, and so on) seems a serious wrong – even though there is no actual harm done to the patient.

One way to express this wrong is by appealing to the concept of dignity. So one can say that in the above example what the nurses did was wrong because she failed to respect the dignity of the patient. We have not mentioned any principle or rule of dignity so far, so what is relationship between dignity and the principles, rules and theories we have heard about so far? I would suggest that the wrong done to the patient in the example can be expressed in terms of the privacy rule. By not covering the patient up, or screening his bed area from the view of others, the privacy of the patient is grossly violated. So one can see how some moral concepts which don't explicitly appear in the principle-based approach can nonetheless be captured by them.

We now turn to the final clause which issues a recommendation that nurses have 'professional indemnity insurance'. This is not so obviously patient-orientated but we can still see that it is bound up with moral principles regarding promotion of patient well-being and avoidance of harm. From the patient's perspective, it seems appropriate to have some form of redress against negligent nurses. So the existence of a legal framework to protect patients seems clearly important. And from the nurse's perspective too, such a framework is of importance. If a nurse makes an innocent mistake and is at risk of prosecution for negligence, it is important that he can access funds for a proper hearing. If a good nurse is forced out of the profession unfairly, in a small way, patient well-being is affected since the range of acts which the nurse would otherwise have undertaken might not now take place. And if the nurse really is a good nurse, it is of course unfair that she should be denied the opportunity to practice.

This discussion helps to illustrate the ways in which the moral principles and rules presented by Beauchamp and Childress are represented in the code, just as they were in the earlier version which informed the previous edition of this book. In fact, just as it is difficult to see how a coherent moral theory could avoid according great significance to the values captured in the principles and rules, the same can be said of a code of conduct for nurses (or for any other groups of health care professionals). This is because the values in the principles are so fundamental to health care provision.

Some values present in the current code might not be easy to subsume within the four principles, in particular those referring to dignity and respect for persons (as distinct from respect for autonomy). However, for what it is worth, my view is that this is done satisfactorily by the strategy outlined earlier (e.g., by construing respect for persons in terms of beneficence, non-maleficence and justice). And one can also subsume dignity in terms of privacy, respect for autonomy, beneficence and non-maleficence.

Conclusion

In this chapter, then, we have described each of the principles in some depth. Much more could be said about each of them, so it cannot be claimed that the discussion here provides an exhaustive account. Nonetheless, the descriptions of them provided should be found adequate for our purposes. More ambitiously, and contrary to the view of Beauchamp and Childress, arguments in support of an 'autonomy-weighted' interpretation of the principles were presented too. The chapter closed by making explicit the close connections between the four principles and the NMC Code. In the next chapter we will be concerned with moral problems arising from conflicts between the obligations referred to by the four principles. To that task we now turn.

Chapter 4

Conflicts between the Principles

In the last chapter, each of the level-three moral principles which figure in Beauchamp and Childress's principle-based approach was considered. Given understanding of the nature of the obligations referred to by these principles, we now move to consider examples of moral dilemmas which arise due to clashes between moral principles. As will be seen, this will take us into discussions of the ethics of truth-telling, decisions not to resuscitate patients, and the more general topics of autonomy and paternalism. Discussion of the ways in which respect for autonomy, and obligations of beneficence and non-maleficence, can conflict with the principle of justice will lead us to consider the issue of the fair allocation of health care resources. For now though, we turn to clashes between respect for autonomy on the one hand, with beneficence and non-maleficence on the other.

Respect for autonomy in conflict with beneficence and non-maleficence

A great many of the moral problems faced by nurses stem from conflicts between obligations of respect for autonomy on the one hand,

and obligations of non-maleficence and beneficence on the other. A common example of such problems arise in situations involving truth-telling.

Truth-telling

Suppose a patient has a terminal condition and that the health care team believe that informing him about the nature of his condition will make him depressed and merely add to his level of suffering. It might also be thought that to tell the patient would remove all hope from him and be so dispiriting to him that his death is effectively hastened by this news. Moreover, telling the patient the truth might adversely affect him in another way. Suppose the prospects of remission or recovery, though very small indeed, are present nonetheless. Telling the truth to the patient may make these even less likely because the patient simply gives up all hope of recovery. Further, suppose the patient's relatives have been informed about the nature of his condition and that they have requested that he not be told. Such a situation might have arisen if the patient has been unconscious for a time.

This case appears to present a clear clash between the principle of respect for autonomy and the principle of non-maleficence. This is because obligations to respect autonomy include the obligation to be truthful to the patient. But obligations of non-maleficence include obligations not to harm the patient. If being truthful will harm the patient by severely distressing them, or worse, then a moral dilemma is presented and has to be responded to.

One might ask what the relation is between truth-telling and the principle of respect for autonomy. It can be shown that there is a clear link between these notions and, hence, that the level-two rule of veracity has its moral foundation in the level-three principle of respect for autonomy. (It may be recalled that the veracity rule refers to obligations to be truthful – see Chapter 2 above.) For example, Rowson writes:

> [If] someone lies to you, he is reducing your capacity to understand your surroundings; and since this capacity is a valuable part of you as a person, he is thus failing to respect you as a person. (1990, p. 19)

Hence, the suggestion here is that as an autonomous person one needs information in order to maximally exercise one's freedom of choice. For example, suppose a friend of yours is a keen supporter of the football club Wycombe Wanderers and that she is unaware of the fact that her team are playing tonight. You, however, know that they are playing tonight and you deliberately keep this information from your friend, even though it would have been easy for you to tell her this in the many conversations you have had with her since learning that the game is to take place. You are fully aware that your friend would like to be given the information, but you keep it from her. In purposely keeping this information from the person, you reduce the number of choices she recognizes as being available to her and thereby inhibit her autonomy. Another, much more serious, example of a clash between obligations to respect autonomy and other principles can arise in the context of decisions not to resuscitate patients. Such patients typically have a very poor prognosis and it is thought that further treatment in the form of resuscitation would not be in the patient's best interests.

DNR ('do not resuscitate') decisions

In October 2007 a joint statement was issued by the BMA, RCN and the UK Resuscitation Council (BMA, 2007). According to this, nurses with sufficient relevant experience can be given the authority to make decisions about whether or not a patient should be resuscitated. In the past, such decisions were taken by medical staff. Also, in the past, it was common practice not to involve patients in decisions about their 'resuscitation status' – decisions regarding whether or not they were to be resuscitated in the event of their having a cardiac arrest.

So consider a situation in which a patient is not involved in discussions concerning her resuscitation status. One reason for not involving her may be because it is thought that such decisions are medical rather than moral. But, if one did think this, it seems easy to show one would be in error. This is because as we saw in Chapter 1, all actions by health care professionals have a moral dimension to them. This is because, as we heard, such acts aim at moral goals, such as relieving suffering, enhancing quality of life and so on. So there are no 'purely medical' decisions if by this it is meant decisions which have no ethical dimension to them.

Further, as we saw in Chapter 3 during the discussion of non-maleficence, it is possible to bring about a person's death by omission, as opposed to commission. It may be that a DNR decision is made about a patient to prevent the need for them to endure further suffering. Deaths brought about in what are judged to be the best interests of a person are plausibly described as a consequence of acts of euthanasia (the bringing about of a good death). One form of euthanasia is passive euthanasia, which involves bringing about a person's death by omission. Evidently, then, DNR decisions implement passive euthanasia since they are decisions to bring about the death of an individual by omission (the omission to act in ways which will prolong the person's life). So, it is reasonable to claim that DNR decisions have a moral dimension to them for the reasons just given. Plainly, medical facts may be relevant to a moral decision – for example, if a person has only a few days to live which will inevitably be spent in great pain. But the point remains that decisions not to resuscitate patients (or, indeed, decisions to resuscitate them) inescapably have a moral dimension (see also Yarling and McElmurry, 1983).

The second type of reason for not involving patients in DNR decisions arises from consideration of the possible harms or psychological distress which might be caused to them as a direct result of such involvement (but see Robertson, 1993). The view here seems to be that obligations of non-maleficence are so great as to outweigh those to respect the autonomy of patients (see Loehy, 1991).

We have seen two types of issues, then, arising from nursing practice, in which there is a conflict between obligations to respect autonomy on the one hand, and obligations of beneficence and non-maleficence on the other. In fact, there are countless other types of situations in which this type of conflict occurs. A brief list might include the following:

- Asking patients to get out of bed or to move when they do not wish to;

- Asking patients to return to a ward when they do not wish to;

- Asking patients to take medication when they do not wish to;

- Trying to prevent a patient from leaving a ward;

- Entering a patient's house without their permission;

- Moving a patient (say, a patient with a severe physical disability) without seeking the patient's views on the matter;

- Feeding or giving medication to a patient against their wishes;

- Trying to wash a patient without their permission, or against their wishes;

- Treating a patient against their wishes;

- Not respecting a patient's wish to keep their prognosis from their close family (when one thinks it is in the best interests of the patient that they know the prognosis); ·
- Trying to prevent a patient from committing suicide; etc.

A high proportion of the moral problems faced by nurses in their interactions with autonomous patients arise from conflicts between the principle of respect for autonomy, on the one hand, and those of beneficence and non-maleficence on the other. It is common to invoke the concept of paternalism in the characterization of such conflicts (Benjamin and Curtis, 1986; Beauchamp and Childress, 2009, p. 206). So we now turn to a discussion of the relationship between autonomy and paternalism.

Autonomy and paternalism

Put roughly, acts which are intended to benefit, or prevent harm befalling another person, but are not at the request of that person, are paternalistic acts. Benjamin and Curtis (1986) favour the term 'parentalism', as opposed to 'paternalism' since the latter may be open to the charge of being sexist: clearly female parents may also act paternalistically, and so parentalism seems the more accurate term here. In spite of this, I will continue to use the term 'paternalism', since 'parentalism' seems not to be in common usage. Benjamin and Curtis characterize paternalistic acts rather memorably as acts in which

> The nurse [or other health care professional] will claim to be acting *on the behalf*, although *not at the behest*, of the patient. (1986, p. 53; also Beauchamp and Childress, 2009, p. 208)

Hence, suppose a nurse intentionally disregards a patient's expressed wishes not to receive pressure-area care; perhaps the patient finds the procedure causes discomfort, finds it embarrassing and a little painful. The nurse continues to turn the patient over, however, and give the pressure-area care in spite of what the patient has said.

The nurse in such a situation seems to be acting in a way which satisfies Benjamin and Curtis's characterization: the nurse is, in her view, acting on behalf of the patient though not at the behest of the patient – the opposite in fact. One can see why a nurse might think it justified to give pressure-area care to a physically frail patient even when the patient has said they don't want to have it. The consequences for the patient of developing a pressure sore could be serious, possibly dangerously so, if it extends the patient's stay in hospital. So a nurse might well think it is so obviously in the best interests of the patient to have the pressure-area care that she ensures the patient receives it, irrespective of the patient's own view on the matter.

A parallel analysis can be given for all the types of situations listed a few paragraphs earlier. The nurse wants to act in accord with what he or she thinks to be in the patient's best interests, in spite of the patient's own views.

The term 'paternalism' is intended to suggest the adoption of a parental, protective attitude towards others – in our case, patients or other health care colleagues. Also, it should be recalled that paternalistic actions are motivated by obligations of beneficence and non-maleficence. Because of this, it needs to be stressed that paternalistic actions are not objectionable *per se*. Critiques of paternalistic actions have led some to suppose that if an act is paternalistic it is necessarily morally unjustified. But this is not so. There may be ethically justified paternalistic acts. Indeed, as just noted, such actions may be motivated by adherence to respectable moral principles. However, given the importance or 'moral weight' accorded to the principle of respect for autonomy in this discussion, it is reasonable to claim, at least, that the onus of justification lies with those who seek to override the autonomy of another person. So in the example just discussed, the onus of justification in such a situation lies with the nurse who overrides the express wishes of the patient in what the nurse judges to be in the best interests of that patient.

It is important to emphasize the position just described: the theoretical stance within nursing ethics being proposed here is that in nursing practice, actions which seek to override the autonomy of a patient stand in need of justification. Hence, the mere fact that an action is perceived by a nurse (or other health care professional) to be for the benefit of a patient, is not, in itself, sufficient justification to warrant adoption of that course of action. Thus, it is being claimed that paternalistic actions stand in need of moral justification.

One further point of clarification is needed before continuing. Recall that for Benjamin and Curtis an action is paternalistic if it is on someone's behalf but not at that person's behest. In each of the examples of paternalistic actions which were offered earlier, the patient was conceived to be conscious, rational and able to make a decision. In cases of this nature, obligations of beneficence and non-maleficence clearly conflict with obligations to respect autonomy. But, consider cases in which, say, a person is unconscious and where the person has expressed no view whatsoever with regard to preferences concerning health care (the person has not left a living will, or 'advance decision', for example).

In cases such as these, there is no evident conflict with the autonomy of the unconscious person since that person is not able to express any preferences; and, we are supposing that the person has not hitherto expressed any preferences regarding health care options. Actions intended to benefit such an unconscious person apparently qualify as paternalistic on Benjamin and Curtis's criterion, since they are for the benefit of the unconscious person but not at their behest. This quite broad characterization of paternalistic acts is in agreement with some modern usage, and will be followed here. (See e.g., Beauchamp and Childress, 2009, p. 209) It should be clear, then, that paternalistic acts are to be construed quite broadly to include acts which are for the benefit of another person. Given this, it seems uncontroversial to point out that acts which benefit persons who are unable to express a view on the matter – unable to express any preferences – are easy to justify from the moral perspective. This follows from our earlier points regarding the obligations of beneficence and non-maleficence which bind nurses. As before, it is presumed that the patient has expressed no prior views regarding preferences for treatment options.

Much more controversial moral problems arise from two kinds of cases. First, cases in which an autonomous patient makes a competent decision to pursue a course of action which, in the view of the nurse, will not benefit the patient and may cause harm to the patient. Examples of such situations include cases where patients refuse medication, refuse to get out of bed, refuse pressure-area care, seek early discharge, take harmful drugs, express intentions to commit suicide, or other forms of self harm, and so on. Moral problems of this nature involve conflicts between obligations of respect for autonomy on the one hand, and those of beneficence and non-maleficence on the other.

The second kind of cases include situations in which it is difficult to determine whether or not the patient is, in fact, competent to make a decision to pursue a course of action which, in the view of the nurse, will not benefit the patient and may be harmful to them. The examples offered in the last paragraph can be cited once more here. The areas of nursing in which situations of this nature arise most frequently, it can be supposed, include nursing children, nursing older confused patients and in the mental health setting. Often in those areas it is extremely difficult to determine whether a patient is indeed competent to make a particular decision.

Given acceptance of the earlier claims regarding the importance of respecting the autonomy of patients, it would follow that in straight-forward clashes between that principle and those of beneficence and non-maleficence, obligations to respect autonomy win out. Though, as will shortly be seen, there are serious problem cases, especially with regard to suicidal and other self-harming patients.

If that theoretical stance is accepted, it would follow, further, that the greater the degree of autonomy and competence of a person, the more difficult it is to justify acting paternalistically – that is, acting in that person's interests as they are conceived of by health care professionals, as opposed to how they are conceived of by the person himself. Having made these points, let us continue.

The question which needs to be addressed is this: can there be paternalistic interventions which are morally justified given both (a) the earlier claims regarding the moral weight attached to autonomy, and (b) that our present concern is specifically with moral problems in which the patient is autonomous and competent to make the relevant choice?

Justifying paternalistic interventions

Benjamin and Curtis (1986) offer three necessary conditions which have to be met in order to justify a paternalistic intervention. They claim that:

> An act of parentalism [is] justified if and only if
> 1. the subject is, under the circumstances, irretrievably ignorant of relevant information, or his or her capacity for rational reflection is significantly impaired (the autonomy condition);
> 2. the subject is likely to be significantly harmed unless interfered with (the harm condition); and
> 3. it is reasonable to assume that the subject will, at a later time, with greater reflection, ratify the decision to interfere by consenting to it (the ratification condition). (1986, p. 57)

Hence, for Benjamin and Curtis, all three conditions must be satisfied in order for a paternalistic action to be morally justified. These will be discussed in turn.

The autonomy condition

If a person is aware of 'relevant information' and if the person is able to reason – is capable of 'rational reflection' – then paternalistic interventions will not be justifiable. In short, if a person is competent to make a decision to pursue a particular course of action, it is not justifiable to prevent them.

It should be repeated that there are no obligations to respect autonomy if a person is exercising that autonomy in a way which will harm others (Mill, 1863, p. 135). If a person enters my room with a gun and expresses an intention to shoot me, I am not obliged simply to respect his autonomous wish to do so. Obligations to respect autonomy can justifiably be overridden when a person seeks to transgress the autonomy of others.

In Benjamin and Curtis's view, for a paternalistic intervention to be justified, it is necessary that the person is not autonomous – more specifically, that the person lacks the competence to make the decision, either through ignorance of relevant information, or intoxication or some other factor affecting their ability to make a decision. This is a very extreme position, and it will be contrasted with an alternative line from Beauchamp and Childress later. Consider now, though, Benjamin and Curtis's 'harm condition'.

The harm condition

By this, for a paternalistic intervention to be justified it is necessary that the patient is open to high risk of 'significant harm'. If no harm is likely to befall the patient, then a paternalistic intervention cannot be justified. Perhaps more seriously, the mere fact that a course of action recommended by a health care professional is likely to benefit a person is not taken to be a sufficient justification for a paternalistic intervention. This position sits well with our earlier points regarding the relative moral weights attached to autonomy and beneficence.

One immediate difficulty with the harm condition appears to be raised by the term 'significant harm'. It seems plausible to suppose that, say, a course of action which will lead to serious injury (loss of a limb, for example), will count as significant harm. Further, it is possible to identify a class of harms which are psychological harms. Severe depression, schizophrenia and other mental health problems which involve distress to their sufferers all seem to be relevant here. Benjamin and Curtis offer only the example of cigarette smoking as an activity which runs a high risk of significant harm (1986, p. 60). Also, as we have seen, it can be difficult to determine just what is the least harmful outcome in cases where differing conceptions of harm are involved.

In spite of difficulties concerning its application, the term 'significant harm' of Benjamin and Curtis might still prove to be worth taking seriously. This, once more, is due to the view that obligations to respect autonomy carry more moral weight than those of non-maleficence. Hence, it is evident that persons capable of competent decisions are not prevented from undertaking many activities which involve a high risk of significant harm. Examples of such activities include smoking, heavy alcohol consumption, excessive consumption of unhealthy foodstuffs, cycling, mountaineering, motor racing, motor cycling, boxing, and so on. Clearly, in the prevailing moral climate autonomous persons (specifically those over the age of 18) are not prevented from undertaking very many potentially harmful courses of action. To accept this position for persons outside the health care context, and to deny it to patients, would be unfair.

To a large extent, then, any worries one has over the extent of the application of the term 'significant harm' can be put to one side in a substantial class of cases. Specifically, cases in which autonomous individuals make competent decisions to engage in types of actions which are harmful to them and to them alone. Indeed, such a position is reflected in the law (see Chapter 3). Competent adults are entitled to refuse even life-saving treatment, and to treat them against their wishes constitutes criminal assault (Mason and McCall Smith, 1994, p. 234; recall again the case of Emma Gough, the mother of twins who was a Jehovah's witness).

So, it is reasonable to accept Benjamin and Curtis's second condition, the harm condition, according to which, for a paternalistic intervention to be justified, it is necessary that the patient will come to significant harm unless the intervention takes place; the risk of minor harm is of course, not enough to justify a paternalistic act. It is important to note that this condition is not a sufficient condition for the justification of paternalistic acts. This is due to the fact that if a patient fails to satisfy the autonomy condition – if he or she is both autonomous and competent – then the fact that that condition is not satisfied indicates that the paternalistic intervention is not justified (since, in effect, Benjamin and Curtis require that a person is not competent before a paternalistic intervention may be taken, see e.g., 1986, p. 57).

The ratification condition

This third condition put forward by Benjamin and Curtis can be illustrated as follows. In the mental health context, it is sometimes the case that patients refuse medication during phases of acute illness. For example, suppose such a patient refuses medication on the grounds that the medication was manufactured by 'devils'. Suppose, further, that the patient is given medication against their wishes – a paternalistic act. As the patient passes through the acute phase of illness towards recovery, it may be that he or she subsequently ratifies the paternalistic actions of the health care team. Perhaps the patients may say that when they look back to the incident when they were given medication against their wishes, they now recognize they were ill at that time and are now, in fact, pleased they received the medication, even though, at the time, they were refusing it.

For another example, consider that a very young child refuses to go to the the dentist in spite of his parents' exhortations (adapted from Benjamin and Curtis, 1986, p. 53). Eventually, the parents coerce the child into visiting the dentist. The child, having now grown up with beautiful teeth, recalls the struggles with his parents caused by the visits to the dentist. Recognizing that his parents were, after all, acting in his best interests, he tells them that he is now pleased they acted against his wishes and coerced him into undergoing dental treatment. In such an example, the child 'ratifies' the paternalistic actions of his parents.

One may feel justifiably suspicious with respect to the ratification condition. It seems to require that health care professionals peer into the future to speculate upon the patient's attitude at a later time to the paternalistic intervention. And of course this is not possible. Also, in many cases one wonders what such speculation could achieve. Nurses may think they know a patient well, but be completely mistaken. As noted in Chapter 1, hospital admission can be a disorientating experience for patients, and they may not behave normally whilst they are in such unusual circumstances. Given that, there is much room for error in attempting to make the kind of assessment required by the ratification condition. If the nurse knows a patient very well, obviously it is more likely that the nurse will have an idea of whether or not the patient would ratify the intervention. But as indicated here, even then there is much scope for doubt about this. When nurses know very little about the values and character of a patient, the grounds for the kind of assessment required by the ratification condition seem extremely insecure. And, because of this, the ratification condition could be open to abuse. This must constitute a grave concern as far as the adoption and application of this condition is concerned.

Having expressed that, quite serious, reservation it does seem that there are circumstances in which it may be feasible to apply the ratification condition in such a way that the possibility of its abuse is minimized. For example, in the context of mental health nursing, it is often the case that nurses build up relationships with patients (and their relatives) which are quite long-standing. A nurse may well feel with good reason that they are in a position to make a judgement about what the patient would want to happen in a particular type of situation. Perhaps, over time, the nurse has come to learn about the patient's attitudes and values. It may even be supposed that certain possible future events have been discussed between the nurse and the patient. For example, suppose a patient has schizophrenia, and that they regularly go through a recognizable cycle of acute breakdown, and medication-sustained recovery. It may be that the nurse could discover during the patient's stable, illness-free periods just what kinds of intervention they would prefer to happen in the event of the onset of an acute phase of the illness. It may be, for example, that the nurse could put to the patient the question: 'In the event of you refusing to take medication at some point in the future (within specified limits), would you prefer your wishes expressed at that future time to be respected, or your wishes now to be respected?' In a situation such as that, it seems, the notion of retrospective ratification may have some reasonable application.

Thus far then, we have considered Benjamin and Curtis's criteria for determining whether or not a paternalistic intervention is justified. In their position, as we saw, all three conditions need to be met before such an intervention is justified. That is to say, a person must meet the following three criteria:

- They must not be competent at the relevant time (the person must meet the autonomy condition);

- It must be the case that the course of action pursued by the person is highly likely to result in significant harm to them (the person must meet the harm condition);

- It must be the case that the person is highly likely to ratify the proposed paternalistic intervention at some later time (the person must meet the ratification condition).

It should be said that given our comments on the concept of competence in Chapter 3 previously, the first condition is perhaps better described as a 'competence condition', since the relevant question concerns the competence of the patient. The second condition has been commented on. With respect to the third, the reservations expressed above concerning its application seem serious; but, as indicated above, in cases where there is a therapeutic relationship of sufficient depth which obtains between the nurse and the person, then a role can be envisaged for the ratification condition. But, in other cases, for example where the wishes of the patient are not known and there are no friends or relatives available to indicate the patient's beliefs and values, then it is hard to envisage a defensible role for the ratification condition. Hence, it does not seem plausible to include satisfaction of the ratification condition in a list of necessary or sufficient conditions relevant to the justification of paternalistic interventions. More plausibly, in certain types of case, a ratification condition may comprise a necessary but not a sufficient condition of justified paternalism.

Given these comments, then, the following conclusion can be advanced. Paternalistic interventions are only justified when the person is not competent. This conclusion is entirely congenial to the general position being tentatively advanced in this book: it is one in which the principle of respect for autonomy is being accorded the greatest of moral weight (due to the considerations advanced in Chapter 3 and in the above discussion of paternalism).

As mentioned, this is a very strong (in the sense of extreme) position to take and so some further comment on it is appropriate. Beauchamp and Childress refrain from supporting such an extreme 'autonomy weighted' position, they state 'we also argue that beneficence sometimes provides grounds for justifiably restricting substantially autonomous actions' (2009, p. 209). As can be seen then, in contrast with Benjamin and Curtis, and the line suggested here, Beauchamp and Childress maintain that paternalistic actions can be justified even when a person is acting autonomously. They outline five conditions, each of which must be satisfied, if such an act is justified. These are:

1. The patient is at risk of a significant, preventable harm. 2. The paternalistic action will probably prevent the harm. 3. The projected benefits to the patient of the paternalistic action outweigh its risks to the patient. 4. There is no reasonable alternative to the limitation of autonomy. 5 The least autonomy-restrictive alternative that will secure the benefits and reduce the risks is adopted. (2009, p. 216)

To illustrate this, here is an example of a paternalistic intervention which would not be justifiable according to the above conditions. A patient with a terminal condition seeks to take an overdose of opiates to end his suffering, which in the view of the patient is pointless in light of his imminent, inevitable death.

To prevent the patient from taking the overdose would, from the moral point of view (which we can insulate from legal considerations for the sake of the discussion here) count as a paternalistic intervention, taken ostensibly in the best interests of the patient or to prevent harm to the patient. However, it would not be a justified one according to the five conditions which Beauchamp and Childress propose. This is because the harm which will befall the patient, the suffering prior to death, is not preventable. Nor is the second condition met since the harm is not prevented. The third condition is more problematic to apply but it looks again as though it will not be met. This is because it is not clear how to assess 'benefits' independently of the patients own assessment of what would, for him, count as beneficial. The fourth condition is not met since there is a 'reasonable alternative' to the limitation of autonomy. This consists in respecting the patient's view and to refrain from preventing him taking the overdose. And lastly, the benefits secured by preventing him from taking the overdose – setting aside problems in determining the assessment of benefit here – probably would count as being the 'least autonomy-restrictive' in one sense. This is because they involve only removing the opiates from the patient's possession and not, instead, say, binding his hands to make it impossible for him to attempt to take the overdose. In another sense, of course, to prevent the patient taking the opiates is indeed grossly 'autonomy-restrictive' in the sense that the patient's own, autonomously chosen, plans for his death are thwarted.

Let us turn now to a more contentious example. This is one offered by Beauchamp and Childress as an example of a *justified* paternalistic act; it thus presents a serious challenge to the position defended so far in this book. The example is from the nursing context and runs as follows:

After receiving his pre-operative medicine, C, a 23 year-old male athlete scheduled for a hernia repair, states that he does not want the side rails up. C is of clear mind and understands why the rule is required; however, C does not feel the rule should apply to him because he is not in the least bit drowsy from the pre-operative medication and he has no intention of falling out of bed. After considerable discussion between the nurse and the patient, the nurse responsible for C's care puts the side rails up. Her justification is as follows: C is not drowsy because he has just received the pre-operative medication, and its effects have not occurred. Furthermore, if he follows the typical pattern of patients receiving this medication in this dosage, he will become very drowsy very quickly. A drowsy patient is at risk for a fall. Since there is no family at the hospital to remain with the patient, and since the nurses on the unit are exceptionally busy, no one can constantly stay with C to monitor his level of alertness. Under these circumstances, the patient must be protected from the potential harm of a fall, despite the fact that he does not want this protection. ... The nurse restricted this autonomous patient's liberty based on ... protection of the patient from potential harm ... and *not* as a hedge against liability or for protection from criticism. (Beauchamp and Childress, 2009, p. 215; the case appeared originally in Silva, 1989)

So this looks like a plausible example of a justified paternalistic act in spite of the fact that the nurse overrides the autonomously expressed views of the patient. To see how this is justified according to their own criteria, recall that the patient is at risk of a 'significant, preventable harm' (ibid.) which would probably be prevented by the paternalistic act; the benefits to the patient outweigh any risks; there is no other 'realistic alternative to the limitation of autonomy'; and this looks like an action which is only minimally restrictive – the patient will soon be too drowsy to get up and in the interim could let down the side rails if distressed by them.

Conversely, by Benjamin and Curtis's analysis (provided the example is taken to constitute one of justified paternalism), it looks like it would not be justifiable to overrule the patient's choice in this case. This is because if the patient is autonomous and makes the competent decision to reject the offer of the side rails being put up, then paternalism cannot be justified. This is the case, for them, even if harm is likely to befall the patient, and even if the patient would later ratify the paternalistic act. As we saw in discussion of Benjamin and Curtis's approach all three conditions need to be met before paternalism is justified.

So, which position in relation to the justification of paternalistic acts is the most defensible? In looking at this question it is important to look again more closely at the example provided by Beauchamp and Childress. Recall that for an action to count as paternalistic, the sole motivation must be to protect the interests of the person concerned – in the example described this is the patient C. Now recall this sentence from the case example 'since the nurses on the unit are exceptionally busy' (ibid.). The clear implication here is that as the nurses are so busy, staying with C to prevent his falling out of bed would jeopardize the levels of care for other patients and may indeed place them in some danger. If this is the sole, or even the primary, justification for raising the side rails on C's bed, then this action is not a paternalistic one. It fails to meet a necessary condition of a paternalistic act, this being that it be 'on the behalf but not at the behest ' (Benjamin and Curtis, 1986, p. 53) of the patient. The main justification for the nurse's act is the safety of all the patients in his or her clinical area of responsibility. And that is perfectly justifiable. But to act from those motivations is not to act paternalistically since the act is motivated by consideration of the interests of parties besides those of C.

A second query about the example is the competence of C to refuse the side rails. His refusal only counts as competent if it is based upon awareness of the dangers of not having the side rails raised. Again, as the example is described it is not clear that C is aware that, although he feels clear-headed at the time of the discussion with the nurse, he will rapidly lose this state of mind. Also, again in relation to the feasibility of the actual example, one imagines that C could actually simply put the side rails down again if he wanted to after the nurse had raised them.

Further, one might think by providing an explanation to the patient of what will happen once he has the pre-operative medication, the problem need not have arisen in the first place.

However, having raised these queries about the example, let us agree, for the sake of argument both (a) that the sole justification for raising the side rails is to protect the interests of C, and does not stem from considerations about the safety of other patients (and staff); and (b) that C is indeed aware of relevant risks and so that his decision is indeed competent. Is the paternalistic intervention now justified?

Provided all considerations related to the interests of other patients are set aside – imagine there are sufficient staff numbers to keep an eye on C – to override C's competent refusal of the side rails seems hard to justify, certainly this is true whilst he is conscious. To see this, recall again the points made about Emma Gough above (the Jehovah's witness patient). As we have seen, competent patients are allowed to refuse even life-saving interventions. Respect for autonomy is given such a high standing in the current legal framework that it not only reflects a moral consensus, but also indicates a moral precedent. If that is true, and given all the previous arguments concerning the priority attached to respect for autonomy, it would be hard to see how the nurse could defensibly override C's well-considered decision in the example under discussion.

It may be replied that there is a vast difference between patients who refuse treatment on religious grounds and those who refuse on other grounds. Thus, it may be said, to treat a Jehovah's Witness patient against his or her religious principles is to do a profound wrong to them ('to damage their *substantial* autonomy interests' as Beauchamp and Childress put it (2009, p. 216).) And that there is no similar kind of wrong that could be done to C in his circumstances. But, in response, it seems sufficient to offer the reminder that refusals of treatment by competent persons are to be respected in law, even if they are not grounded in any religious tradition. So, it looks again as though the decision to override C's wish is not justified.

It may be complained that the strategy just offered against paternalism in C's case reduces a moral argument to a legal one, and so is beside the point. However, as Beauchamp and Childress themselves point out, responses to moral problems need to take into account relevant empirical considerations and it seems to me that the legal point just made is one such relevant empirical consideration. Laws do not appear in a moral vacuum, they often reflect a moral consensus – the change in the abortion laws in the both the United Kingdom (1967) and the United States of America (1973) comprise examples of such links between laws and consensus in the common morality. To concede this much to the law is not, of course, to argue that ethical problems can always be resolved satisfactorily by turning to the relevant laws. There may be laws which are immoral, so what is legal may differ from what is moral.

A further response takes a different form. This consists in pointing to a wide range of apparently 'autonomy restricting' practices which, consensus suggests, are morally defensible. Thus, the 'autonomy-weighted' position must imply the overturning of these too, or accept that such positions are justified because of the moral consensus they reflect. The kinds of examples which are relevant here are those such as seatbelt legislation, regarding the compulsory use of motor cycle crash helmets, and against use of mobile phones by drivers whilst they are driving. In the United Kingdom at least it is illegal to do any of these things. How is it possible to reconcile the claim that respect for autonomy is the most weighty moral principle with an acceptance of these practices?

The response to this is as follows. Recall from our discussion of respect for autonomy that obligations to respect it are not without limit. When people exercise their autonomy in ways which impugn the autonomy of others, then there is no obligation to respect the autonomy of the 'impugner'. Recall too the discussion of C above. If C insists on a nurse staying with him until he becomes drowsy, or until he leaves the ward for the operating theatre, because of the shortage of nursing staff on the ward, to respect his request would be to expose others to harms, harms that, given the choice, they would rather not be exposed to. These examples support the claim that the justification for autonomy-limiting legislation rests upon the view of such behaviours adversely affecting the autonomy of others. To see this, it is plausible to claim that legislation of the kind described above prevents avoidable restrictions on the autonomy of the majority. This is because if motor cyclists ride without helmets, or drivers drive without seatbelts they are more likely to cause accidents and so impugn the autonomy of others directly in that way. In causing more casualties to occur, they cause more expenditure on health and, similarly, impact upon autonomy more indirectly by generating a need for increased health spending, which will be generated through increased taxation. So even when broached 'head on' so to speak, it seems to me that Beauchamp and Childress's example does not constitute one of justified paternalism. Nonetheless, the case is a difficult one. Suppose the nurse respects the patient's wish and leaves the side rails down. This is justified, as we have seen, given the weight attached to respect for autonomy. Suppose now, the patient falls unconscious as the medication takes hold. If there are enough staff to enable the nurse to stay with the patient, then the nurse can do so, thus respecting the patient's wish. If there are not sufficient staff, and it really is likely that the patient will fall, then it seems justified to put the side rails up. To do this is not to harm the patient and the nurse is available to care for other patients too as she is required to. Thus either the interests of others enter into the justification for putting up the side rails in this case, and so we do not have a case of paternalism; or, if there are sufficient staff levels, the nurse can stay with the patient to ensure does not fall out of bed.

But let us raise another kind of situation which provides, perhaps, an even sterner test for the kind of 'autonomy-weighted' line being put forward here. This is provided by situations in which people want to end their own lives.

Suicidal people

It needs to be made explicit that the position arrived at here implies that it is not possible to justify preventing a person from committing suicide who has made a competent decision to do so. In fact, in the position tentatively endorsed here it is not possible justifiably to prevent any competent person from harming themselves. Rightly, those from other theoretical perspectives express concern about such a position (as should all proponents of an autonomy-weighted, principle-based approach). It seems excessively harsh and uncaring to state baldly that a competent person should not be prevented from committing suicide. Hence, it is necessary to offer some views on this extremely difficult and distressing issue.

Rational decisions to commit suicide

A first position to be set aside here is the view that anyone who decides to end their own life must be sufficiently mentally unwell that they cannot competently make such a decision, and, hence, that paternalistic interventions are always justified in such cases. In response to such a view, it is worth considering a case example offered by Bloch and Heyd (1981, p. 198). They describe the case of a 65-year-old man who has cancer of the colon with 'widespread secondaries'. He has only a few weeks left to live and states: '[He] would rather die "with dignity" and in full possession of his senses than in excruciating pain which calls for massive doses of narcotic drugs.' The man seeks to acquire a 'sufficient number of hypnotic pills' in order to end his own life – in the way in which he wants it to end. (See also Voluntary Euthanasia Society, 1992; now 'Dignity in dying' www.dignityindying.org.uk).

The clear implication of Bloch and Heyd's discussion is that it is indeed perfectly rational for the person they describe to decide to commit suicide. His remaining few weeks of life promise only continued suffering and inevitable death. It seems entirely rational, given such terrible prospects, to desire to avoid that avoidable and pointless period of suffering. The VES publication referred to in the last paragraph contains descriptions of similar, equally distressing case examples.

Given acceptance of the claim that there can be suicidal acts which are rational – that result from competent decisions to do so – it needs to be made explicit that it does not thereby follow that all suicidal acts are rational. It is evident that a person's suicidal feelings may well result from a transient mood or mental health problem. Indeed, certain kinds of mental health problems are particularly associated with the risk of suicide (e.g., depression, schizophrenia and alcoholism).

It is useful to draw attention to a continuum of types of cases. At one end we find those in which an autonomous person makes a competent decision to end their own life. Perhaps the example provided by

Bloch and Heyd above constitutes such a case. At the other end is to be found cases in which the person is not autonomous and is clearly not competent to decide to take his or her own life. Perhaps a person is in the acute phase of schizophrenia and wishes to end her life due to the perceived presence of a venomous snake in her stomach. In between these two poles of the continuum there is a variety of much more difficult types of cases in which it is not clear to what degree the person is competent to make a decision to commit suicide. Given what was said earlier in relation to paternalistic acts, it should be clear that justifying such interventions is much less problematic in the cases where the person's decision is not competent and, also, even where the person's competence is in doubt.

In cases of the kind described by Bloch and Heyd above, it is relatively easy to appreciate that the decision made by the patient is a rational one, when the future promises only certain death and pain. It is plausible that paternalistic interventions designed to prevent such a person from committing suicide are extremely hard to justify. Certainly, employing the schema of Benjamin and Curtis (1986), such a person would seem to meet none of the conditions they identify as necessary for the justification of paternalistic interventions. The person fails to satisfy the autonomy condition; the person will come to significant harm whether prevented or 'permitted' to end his own life; and it is extremely unlikely, given the person's reasons for committing suicide, that he would later ratify actions designed to prevent him from taking his own life.

Much more difficult cases are those in which a person wishes to end his own life on the grounds that the future appears to promise a greater amount of suffering than of pleasure, and so decides to end life now rather than endure the anticipated suffering (see Hewitt and Edwards, 2006). Such a person decides that life is simply not worth living or is 'tired of life' (Berghmans and Widdershoven, 2007). It is not hard to envisage circumstances in which a person might well consider suicide on the basis of the likelihood that life has little to offer. Indeed, Camus claims that 'All healthy men [and women] have thought of their own suicide' (1955, p. 13). It is certainly the case that persons other than those suffering from a terminal illness, or extremely debilitating health problem, seriously consider suicide. Given this, an autonomy-weighted position implies that it is not justifiable to prevent such a person from taking his own life. This conclusion seems sufficiently jarring to warrant further attention: it seems that emotional factors seek to override logical conclusions here. This is, indeed, a commonly voiced criticism of the principle-based approach, and one which will be returned to in Chapter 5.

In his discussion of suicide, Harris (1985) seems adamant that persons who make competent decisions to end their own lives cannot justifiably be prevented from doing so (Harris, 1985, p. 203). But Glover in his discussion (1977, chapter 13) and Bloch and Heyd (1981) are less sure. For example, Bloch and Heyd point to a special, perhaps unique, feature of suicidal acts, namely their irreversibility (1981, p. 200). They identify an asymmetry between decisions not to prevent a suicidal act, and decisions to prevent such an act. Obviously, if a suicidal act is successfully undertaken, there are no opportunities available for the suicidal person to reconsider his views. But, if a person is prevented from committing suicide, then such an opportunity is made available. This asymmetry may be taken to support a position in which it is justifiable to prevent a person committing suicide – at least to give the person more time to consider his views. Glover suggests, in fact, that it is 'always legitimate' (1977, p. 176) to reason with a person who expresses suicidal intentions. He claims that such an intervention does not amount to a violation of respect for autonomy. Further, perhaps surprisingly, he claims that it is legitimate to 'restrain by force' (1977, p. 177) a person who is not persuaded against suicide by rational means. The view seems to be that if a person is sufficiently determined to take his own life, then he can simply do so at a future date.

So, the paternalistic stance apparently endorsed by Glover and by Bloch and Heyd, stems from the claim that due to the special nature of suicidal actions – the asymmetry between intervention and non-intervention – the general obligations to respect autonomy can be overridden. This position clearly deserves sympathy, but there are difficulties in resting so much on the claimed asymmetry between decisions to intervene to prevent suicide, and decisions not to intervene. Other examples of irreversible actions may include giving away all one's property, and possibly other types of acts such as donating a kidney, but, these would not be of the same gravity as suicidal acts.

However, attaching such weight to irreversibility may not, in the end, be plausible. This is because at least two counter arguments are available. First, it can be argued that the appeal to irreversibility is simply a red herring. The moral dilemma raised by suicidal intentions stems from a conflict between respect for autonomy and other moral principles (non-maleficence for example); this is the real issue, it may be argued. Hence, the irreversibility or otherwise of suicidal acts is wholly irrelevant to the question of whether it is ethically justifiable to intervene to prevent suicide. Second, one might go further and put forward the view that the very fact that suicidal acts are irreversible, renders them of such significance that they should simply be left to the actor. This response 'turns the tables' so to speak against Bloch and Heyd's argument. The idea of irreversibility may be appealed to in support of the view that since such decisions are so momentous in the life of the person, they should be left with that person and not interfered with. So, it seems not to be the case that much mileage can be gleaned from Bloch and Heyd's suggestion – at least as far as the present author can discern; and, hence, that paternalistic interventions are no easier to justify in relation to suicidal people than they are in people whose actions present other types of moral problems. Given this rather uncomfortable conclusion, let us now move on to consider conflicts between respect for autonomy and the principle of justice.

Autonomy in conflict with justice: allocation of scarce resources

These conflicts arise when autonomous requests for health care resources are frustrated by unavailability of the relevant resource. Thus, suppose a frail person, Mr Jones, who lives alone, finds himself in need of some basic home help support. Mr Jones finds it difficult to cope with going to the shops and his mobility is deteriorating rapidly too. With some home support he would be able to continue to live in his own home but without it, he will need to consider a move into sheltered accommodation, or even a nursing home. Mr Jones's community nurse is very concerned that Mr Jones's health will deteriorate rapidly unless he receives sufficient home support. If there were sufficient resources to support Mr Jones in his own home, he would be able to stay there. As it turns out, there are not enough resources to support him safely at home and he moves to a nursing home. When asked, he says he would much prefer to be at home with some home support in place.

In this example, respect for the autonomy of Mr Jones in his preferred way would require the provision of the kind of home support that he wants. But, if it is not possible to provide such support due to resource shortages, then it is not possible to respect his autonomous request about this issue. Moreover, the reason is due solely to the absence of the resources needed to satisfy the request. This is an example of the way in which obligations to respect autonomy can clash with those of justice. In this example, the relevant budget is distributed amongst the relevant population in such a way that it is not possible to fund the level of support needed if Mr Jones stays in his own home.

Another, even more stark illustration of the way in which autonomy clashes with justice concerns the availability of donor organs. Suppose there are ten patients in need of a kidney transplant and who could be matched perfectly to an available kidney. In such a situation there are ten requests for the resource – the kidney – but only one person can receive it. Assume each could derive an equal level of benefit from the kidney, and there is no other apparent way to distinguish between them in terms of their entitlement to receive the kidney. Again, here, there is a clash between obligations to respect autonomy and those of justice. Sometimes it is simply not possible to meet all autonomous requests for a scarce resource, as the kidney example shows. But what would be a fair way to allocate resources, given that it is not possible to respect all autonomous requests for such?

Before turning to address this question it is worth making explicit the point that it is not simply obligations to respect autonomy that can come into conflict with those of justice. To see this note how obligations of beneficence are apparently thwarted in this hypothetical example. Suppose a decision is made to ensure that all those people with severe intellectual disabilities who are currently cared for at home by, for example, their relatives are to be given the option of having 24-hour individual care – in addition to the care currently given by their relatives. The care would be provided by specially trained care workers.

It is reasonable to suppose that this scheme would improve the lot of those who opt to take it up. If asked to justify such a scheme, the minister for health concerned could remind her questioners of the obligations of beneficence that her decisions are informed by. So the scheme looks prima facie justified on the grounds that the well-being of those who receive it will be increased. And we can assume, reasonably enough, that their levels of well-being would indeed be enhanced by the implementation of the scheme.

But opponents of the scheme might point to the high cost of it, and say that such expenditure could be used in other ways, ways which might lead to greater benefits for a much greater number of patients.

This illustrates the way in which obligations of beneficence are also 'bump up against' those of justice. A decision not to pursue the scheme would display a different set of priorities. A decision to pursue it would manifest a set of priorities that differ from those employed to try to overturn it. There comes a point at which, even though people with health problems could benefit from more resources being given to them, such resources are not forthcoming. Typically, this is because they are distributed to address the health problems of a different group. But what this illustrates is the way in which obligations of beneficence too can conflict with those of justice. Most of us would agree that it would not be a fair way to distribute resources in such a way that a small minority received a very great benefit, whilst the rest suffered.

Such arguments manifest differing opinions about the fairest ways to allocate health care resources. Four criteria may be proposed concerning the fair allocation of health care resources. These are that health care resources should be allocated: according to need; according to desert; according to right; and according to utility; these criteria may be referred to, respectively, as needs-based, desert-based, rights-based, and utility-based criteria (see Gillon, 1985).

Before moving on to consider these four criteria, other points of clarification are required. First, how is the term 'allocation' to be understood in questions concerning resource allocation? It is customary to draw a distinction between macroallocation, mesoallocation, and microallocation of health care resources (Gillon, 1985, chapter 15). Rather crudely, questions of macroallocation concern the proportion of the finances available to a government which is to be allocated to health care – as opposed to, say, arms and education. Microallocation of resources is said by Gillon to involve decisions such as choosing between 'competing claimants' (1985, p. 93) for, say, a kidney dialysis machine or a place in a special care baby unit. And mesoallocation concerns questions of distribution of resources between the macro and micro-levels (say at the level of an NHS Trust regarding the spending of its budget).

From the specifically nursing perspective, it can be pointed out that nurses are perpetually making decisions concerning the way they should divide the time they spend with patients. Of course, nursing time is itself a health care resource (Dickenson, 1994). A community nurse with a large case-load has to decide which is the fairest way to manage it. Inevitably, less time will be allocated to certain patients than to others. But which criteria will the nurse employ in order to make such a decision?

Similarly, in a ward situation, a nurse may be aware that there is only a limited supply of clean bed linen available for the patients she is directly responsible for. How should she decide which patients will receive clean linen, and which ones will have to make do? (Assuming that simply walking away in protest is not an option – see Chapter 7.) So, nurses evidently have to make decisions at the level of microallocation, and probably at the level of mesoallocation also in so far as they may be involved in such decision-making at the level of the relevant trust management board. But, further, the NMC Code (2008; see Appendix) appears to require that nurses concern themselves with the values which inform macroallocation of health care resources. This is because it refers to an obligation to 'protect and promote the health and wellbeing of...the wider community' (NMC, 2008; see Appendix). So if a nurse becomes aware that a group of people are having difficulties accessing services they are in need of, this aspect of the code seems to suggest that the nurse should try to do something to remedy the situation. If the relevant group are suffering because of some aspect of health policy which is decided at Government level, it seems to follow that the code obliges nurses concerned to try to change such policies so that the needs of the neglected group are addressed properly. This issue is returned to at the end of the present section.

By way of further clarification, it should be noted that health care ranges from care given in the hospital setting, to care given in the community, in addition to health education and promotion. And resources should be taken to include personnel (medical, nursing, administrative, ancillary, and so on), equipment, research findings, research projects, and buildings necessary for the implementation of health care. Having made these preliminary points, let us now move on to look at the four criteria suggested above in answer to the question of what is the fairest way to allocate health care resources. As will be seen, all four criteria provide a different answer to the question. Yet it is true that they all respect the formulation of justice given in Chapter 3 according to which a distribution is just if and only if equals are treated equally and unequals treated unequally in proportion to relevant differences between them (Beauchamp and Childress, 2009, p. 242). Thus as we will see, a distribution based upon determining entitlement to treatment in terms of utility will hold that justice is done if equals (in terms of utility) are treated equally (either granted or denied treatment) and unequals (in terms of utility) are treated unequally (are responded to differently on grounds of utility). The same applies to the other three criteria. The first one to be considered is a utility-based criterion, according to which resources should be distributed in such a way that they maximize utility.

Utility-based criteria (specifically, social utility)

Applied to Gillon's example of a case involving competing claimants for a kidney dialysis machine, a utility-based criterion would determine that the machine should go to the person whose continued survival would generate the greatest amount of (social) utility. So a just distribution is one which maximizes the greatest amount of social utility. And also that health policies in general should be developed in such a way that they are directed to generate the greatest amount of social utility. This would entail directing resources to those groups and individuals whose continued health is predicted to generate the greatest amounts of social utility and away from other groups and individuals. A rationale for such a policy is indicated in this quote from Rescher:

> [In] its allocation [of health care resources] society 'invests' a scarce resource in one person as against another and is thus entitled to look to the probable prospective 'return' on its investment. (Rescher, quoted in Beauchamp and Childress, 1989, p. 299)

A first question to be asked concerns the term 'returns', how should this be understood? It would be reasonable to construe these in material terms, for example, in terms of how much it is predicted that a person could contribute to the economic development of the relevant society, or whether he or she has children whose potential to contribute to the particular society would be enhanced by the continued survival of the person. This is a reasonable interpretation of the term 'returns' since the 'investments' themselves are bound to be financial ones to cover the costs of educating nurses and doctors, providing needed equipment, buildings, and so on.

It seems plausible that allocation of health care resources along these lines would inevitably favour younger people at the expense of older people, especially much older people, since it seems more likely that the former will have dependants, and that they will be employed, and so contribute to the income generation of society.

As might be anticipated, utility-based criteria can be subjected to a number of criticisms. First, as noted above, it seems that the criterion contains an inbuilt bias towards the young and the economically productive. Apart from objections on other grounds, it may be the case that the citizens of such a society come to recognize that they are only valued when they are economically productive, or young. In the light of this, they may decide to go and live elsewhere in a society which has other values. So it is possible that application of the (social) utility-based criterion may turn out to result in a longer-term disutility.

Second, a query arises relating to the consistency of the utility-based view. Recall the quote from Rescher offered earlier. Might not an older person who has contributed taxes to the state during a lengthy working life claim that *he* is entitled to a 'return' on his investment?

Third, it would seem to follow from the adoption of a social utility criterion that, say, a 35-year-old person who arrives in a particular country never having previously visited there, nor contributed anything to the country by payment of taxes, would have a greater chance of receiving scarce resources than a person who has paid taxes for 50 years and is now aged 80. This offends intuitive views of justice as 'desert' (cf. Chapter 3).

Fourth, cases in which there is a clear contrast between the respective utility of two candidates for resources can mask difficulties in the utility-based view. Such difficulties can be exposed by consideration of other types of case. For example, suppose a 25-year-old person and a 26-year-old person are competing for scarce resources; also that they are each in need of similar care, and have similar qualifications, skills, and so forth. It seems simply arbitrary from the moral perspective to claim that the resource should go to the younger person on the grounds that that person has more opportunities (one extra year) to contribute to the economy of the relevant society.

And generally, allocation of health care resources based on social utility alone seems open to many of the standard difficulties which dog Utilitarianism; these include difficulties in predicting consequences of actions, riding roughshod over the autonomy of people, exposing the vulnerable to risk of neglect, and so on. In light of the weaknesses of a utility-based approach, consider an allocation based upon respecting the rights of potential patients.

A rights-based criterion

According to this view, health care resources go to those who have a right to them. The plausibility of this view stems in part from the increasingly widespread employment of appeals to rights. One hears of the rights of the unborn child, the rights of women over their own bodies, rights to health care, to privacy, to education, to free speech, to silence, to information, and so on. And, of course, the now almost forgotten *The Patient's Charter* (Department of Health, 1991) was one attempt to anchor claims relating to provision of health care resources in the language of rights. More recently, the policy document *Human Rights in Health Care – a Framework for Local Action* (Department of Health, 2007) tries a similar thing. So, perhaps in contrast to the idea of a policy for distribution of resources based solely upon considerations of social utility, approaches grounded in rights are very easy to locate and are well supported.

There seem good reasons for this. The articulation of claims to health care resources in terms of rights seems a legitimate extension of appeals to rights which are already well established. Thus claiming a right to fertility treatment or to an expensive cancer treatment seems in the same moral domain as claims about rights to free speech or to religious freedom or to political representation, and so on. Extending appeals to rights to claims to health care resources seems a strong 'tactical' manoeuvre on the part of those who seek such resources but are denied them. Describing such denials as a denial of a *right* seems, at least, a powerful rhetorical claim.

The presentation of a claim to health care resources as a claim to something one has a right to also seems to require at least a response from those upon one whom is making the claim (typically the local NHS Trust). This is because, if they do not respond, their failure to do so can be framed as a failure to give a justification for denying someone a service to which they have a right. Relatedly, such appeals can usefully highlight gaps in health care provision, thus for example if it is shown that wards are not being kept clean the 'wrong' done because of this can be articulated as a violation of patients' right to be cared for in clean and hygienic conditions (see 'The ward smelt of diarrhoea' BBC, 11/10/07). And, perhaps most importantly, since there seems wide agreement about some very basic rights (to free speech, privacy etc.), these can be appealed to to protect the interests of patients. Thus the DoH document referred to above bases the involvement of patients in decisions about their care in a 'Right to respect for private life' (Department of Health , 2007, p. 14). So, basic ethical aspects of the relationships between health care professionals and patients are described as being founded upon widely agreed moral norms such as rights to respect and to privacy.

Evidently, then, an attempt to distribute health care in such a way that those with a right to it have that right met would be thought attractive by many. But is the claim that a fair distribution is one based solely on a duty to respond to rights plausible? This would involve treating equals equally, and unequals unequally so that those with an equal right to health care resources are responded to in the same way; as are those with an unequal right to such care. Thus, if two persons have the same right to resource X (an expensive cancer drug), such a distribution would entail they are responded to in the same way – either both receive the drug or both are denied it. Or, if some *relevant* difference between them can be shown (perhaps one will benefit more than the other) then it could be fair to give the drug to one but not the other. This is, of course, what is involved in 'treating unequals unequally' they are unequal in the sense that one will benefit from the drug more than the other.

To begin to appreciate any such rights-based approach it is important to draw attention to two distinct types of rights; those which make demands upon material resources, and those which do not. Rights of the first kind would include rights to education and to health care, for example. Clearly, in order for it to be possible for these rights to be met, certain material conditions have to be in place. For rights to health care to be met, it follows that the resources necessary to provide that care need to be in place; similarly, with rights to education, shelter, and food. A different type of rights do not seem so obviously dependent upon the availability of material resources – perhaps a right to free speech is an example.

Rights of the first kind are described by Beauchamp and Childress as 'positive rights' (2009, p. 352): these invoke the 'right to receive a particular good or service from others'. Hence, rights to health care resources are plausible examples of positive rights. They include for example, the right to receive certain benefits such as emergency treatment in an Accident and Emergency Unit, or to access a General Practitioner or Community Nurse, or Practice Nurse, or rights to treatments such as IVF, or cancer care or in fact any other intervention which uses some health care resource. Negative rights do not necessarily require any such resources from third parties. All these rights require is that one is left alone, that one's personal sphere is not intruded upon unjustly.

The reason the distinction between positive and negative rights is important is this. The category of negative rights – rights to be left alone and not be interfered with – does not imply the availability of material resources to meet them. To respect someone's privacy is to leave them alone if that is what they want. As we have seen, respecting a right such as this is entirely different from respecting a right to receive health care due to the resources required in claims regarding the latter. A danger in the appeals to rights is that because the kinds of rights expressed by negative rights are so compelling, it is then inferred that they have the same weight when rights are claimed as positive rights. But, it is open to us to accept that people have negative rights and that it is the duty of others to respect these, but at the same time deny there is any similar weighty moral duty to respect positive rights. To illustrate: my rights of privacy entail that nobody can force me to eat cream cakes, I have a negative right to refuse cream cakes; but it would not be plausible to think it follows from this that I have a right to *receive* cream cakes. To think that it did would be a mistake.

So it is indeed coherent to recognize the importance and moral weight of negative rights without being persuaded by the view that positive rights have a similar moral weight. Thus one can reject the view that a fair distribution of health care resources is one grounded in responding to rights to such resources without, at the same time, abandoning commitment to respect for rights such as privacy, free speech, respect, and so on. This point helps to deflate some of the rhetorical force that appeals to rights can have because to deny that someone has a 'right' to an expensive cancer drug is not necessarily morally on a par with denying they have rights to free speech, privacy, and other negative rights.

Consider some difficulties in employing a rights-based criterion. First, in cases of the kind referred to by Gillon (1985) – namely, those which involve equally legitimate claims on limited resources (kidney machines, special-care baby unit places) – the appeal to rights seems entirely redundant. If only one machine or bed is available, the unlucky person may appeal to her right to receive the treatment, but it does not follow from this that she will receive it. The same is true when two people claim the same right to any treatment of limited availability.

Second, given the distinction between negative and positive rights, one can see that there is risk of a kind of vacuity in speaking about positive rights. To see this, imagine a military dictator of a poor country in which there is little or no health care provision. He declares that all his citizens have a right the best health care. Obviously, such a claim is meaningless since there are no provisions available to meet such rights.

A third kind of difficulty arises when one attempts to assess which rights are the most weighty. Given a limited health care budget, priorities in health care spending have to be set. Suppose it is agreed that all citizens have a right to be cared for in their own homes should they or their partner want this. At the time of writing, the Alzheimer's society in the United Kingdom are campaigning for better care for people with

Alzheimer's disease who are in care homes. In the story 'Care staff sedated him by 4.00 p.m.' (BBC,. 27/11/07), Connie Harris, the wife of Lionel Harris who has Alzheimer's describes the poor care her husband received at a care home. The care was so bad she brought him back home. It is plain from the article that she would prefer him to be at home but cannot cope without very considerable levels of support. Suppose she, on behalf of her husband, claims that his rights to a proper level of health care are being violated; so too are the rights of the many other people with the same disease. If one adopts a rights-based criterion of allocation, how can one compare a claim made of this kind against a claim made, for example, to an expensive cancer treatment? Or to free IVF cycles?

As a further illustration of this problem, an influential campaign led to a widening of the availability of the breast cancer treatment drug Herceptin. But recently an expert in the field of radiotherapy claimed that re-directing the same level of expenditure from Herceptin towards radiotherapy would benefit far more patients. The figures given were as follows: in 2006 the NHS spent £100million on Herceptin, which 500 patients benefited from. It was claimed that investing the same amount of money into radiotherapy facilities would benefit far more patients – 30,000 as opposed to only 500 ('Call to redirect cancer drug cash', BBC, 29/11/07). This is a further example of the way in which the expression of claims to health care in terms of rights can lead to a skewing of the distribution of resources in favour of those who articulate such rights most effectively.

As seen, the framing of these problems of fair distribution in terms of violations of rights does not lend itself to a way of assessing whose rights should count for the most. All we seem left with are competing rights claims. We know that not all can be met but it seems impossible to find a way forward which is based solely on appeals to rights, but which will be feasible to implement. (I am assuming a finite health budget.)

Given these problems with appeals to rights, one might reasonably try to argue that the idea of health care *needs* provides a more promising option upon which to base a fair distribution of health care resources.

A needs-based criterion

According to this criterion, resources should go to those who need them – independently of any appeals to rights. On the face of it, this seems an intuitively plausible answer. If a person needs a health care resource, then they should be given it. In fact, *The Patient's Charter* (Department of Health, 1991, p. 8) seems to state a commitment to a needs-based criterion. According to it, 'Every citizen has the [right] to receive health care on the basis of clinical need, regardless of ability to pay'. And much more recently the DoH floated the idea that 'The NHS will provide a universal and comprehensive service with equal access for all, free at the point of use, based on clinical need, not ability to pay' (Department of Health, 2006). The important point for our purposes is the prominence of the idea of clinical need and the implication that this should be the basis of an entitlement to NHS health care resources. Note that this statement is presented as a 'core principle' as opposed to a right (see also Daniels, 1985).

So this kind of approach would entail that a fair distribution would still be one in which 'equals are treated equally, and unequals unequally' but in which the assessment of what counts as being 'equal' is made in terms of needs. Thus two equally needy patients could expect to be treated equally in a distribution of this kind. And two patients who had different levels of health care need could expect to be treated differently (unequals would be treated unequally). An example of the latter kind of distribution would be this.

A nurse is changing a dressing with one patient, when another collapses after walking past. The nurse leaves the patient she had been attending to to go and help the patient that has collapsed. Such an action would still be a fair distribution of her time if the distribution of it is made in terms of meeting needs. For the two patients were 'unequals' in terms of their 'neediness', the needs of the collapsed patient outweigh those of the patient whose dressing is being changed, on this occasion.

Also, this example helps to illustrate a way in which health care needs might be categorized in terms of importance. Thus it may be argued that there is a stronger obligation to meet needs which greatly disrupt a person's capacity to pursue their life plan than to meet needs which disrupt capacity to pursue a plan to a much lesser extent. So someone with peritonitis has a greater health care need than someone with a minor cut. This follows because if left untreated the peritonitis is likely to cause the death of the patient, whilst the patient with the minor cut is in no such danger. (For an interesting attempt to base the distribution of health care on health care needs, see Daniels (1985).)

So can the proposal that a fair distribution is one that is based upon meeting health care needs withstand critical scrutiny? There seem some serious difficulties with such a view. An initial difficulty arises since, clearly, no geographical boundaries are set in the criterion as it stands. To claim simply that resources should go to those who need them, involves setting no criteria for the determination of eligibility to the resources other than 'clinical need'. But, typically, it will be asserted that national boundaries affect one's entitlement to the relevant resources and, hence, that priority will be given to members of a particular society. So, the needs-based criterion, more properly, should be taken to claim that within a specified parameter X, resources should go to those who need them (where 'X' stands for a national, or economic boundary).

A further difficulty for the needs-based view stems from problems distinguishing needs from mere wants. For example, Seedhouse proposes that in matters of health care provision, 'basic needs [should be met] before any other want' (1988, p. 132). For this claim to mean much we need, at least, a definition of the term 'need'. Beauchamp and Childress write 'To say that a person needs something is to say that without it the person will be harmed or at least detrimentally affected' (2009, p. 242). This may be a little too weak, however. A child may genuinely think they are harmed by being denied an expensive toy they want, yet this could count as a need on the description offered by Beauchamp and Childress. It is plausible that whatever needs are, they would at least be caused by a life-threatening condition: the person in such a condition has many health care needs or their life will end. Medical conditions such as cardiac disease, peritonitis, and pneumonia place their sufferers in need of medical treatment. One might attempt to contrast those in need of treatments for such conditions with those who merely *want* or have a desire for some kind of medical intervention – say, infertility treatment, counselling, psychotherapy or cosmetic surgery. But this intuitive division comes under threat since, it seems, any want or desire can be transformed into a need. This follows since a person may claim to be suicidal if denied access to interventions of the kind just referred to. Hence, in this way, a needs-based criterion can seem too weak since it could include interventions usually regarded as mere wants.

In a different way, a needs-based criterion can seem too strong. This is due to the temptation to take a strong line and argue that anything one can live without is a mere want and is not a need. Thus, needs would cover only life-threatening conditions. To see that this is too strong, one need only consider interventions such as eye operations which restore an individual's sight (say, cataract removal), and hip replacements. Each of these types of interventions bestow high levels of opportunities for quality of life improvement on their recipients; also, they are relatively inexpensive procedures. So, it would be implausible to exclude interventions such as these on the basis of the fact that they are not life-threatening.

Further, a needs-based view is vulnerable to one of the same objections which besets a rights-based view; namely, how to cope with situations in which equally needy people require a scarce resource. Evidently, the needs-based criterion is as redundant here as is the rights-based criterion.

So, a commitment to meeting health care needs from a needs-based perspective seems open to at least three substantial objections. There is a problem in specifying just who is potentially entitled to the relevant resources: is it restricted to residents of a specific country or not? Then there is the apparent difficulty that any want can be transformed into a need. Also, there is a temptation to try to ground a distinction between wants and needs by appeal to the life-threatening nature, or otherwise, of specific medical conditions. But this can make the needs-based line far too strong, in that it excludes interventions such as cataract operations and hip replacements. Let us then turn to a different kind of criterion, one based upon what people deserve.

A desert-based criterion

Obviously enough, according to this criterion, health care resources go to those who deserve them. In Gillon's example, the machine would go to the person who had done most to deserve it. In terms of our formal principle of justice, this would entail that equals would be treated equally when those who are equally deserving receive or are denied the relevant resource, and unequals would be treated unequally in the sense that if one person is more deserving of a resource than another, then the resource will go to that person.

Basing decisions about the allocation of health care resources on the idea of who deserves to receive them plainly raises the question of what kinds of activities a person needs to perform in order to be said to deserve health care resources? Here are some suggestions.

- One answer may be that a person must have performed certain types of positively regarded actions, for example, actions which have benefited one's country. These may include fighting for one's country, developing a solution to a serious national problem such as a common disease, or contributing to one's country in some other way, such as by working in the nursing or medical professions.

- A less demanding construal of desert may require merely that the person concerned has contributed financially to the nation's health budget by way of payment of taxes.

- A still less demanding construal would be one in which desert is construed negatively, so to speak. Hence, rather than require that individuals have performed certain types of act, it may be said that persons are entitled to health care resources providing they have *abstained from* specified types of actions. For example, it may be proposed that one is entitled to health care resources providing one has not done anything to render one undeserving of these resources. Examples of actions which may render one undeserving may include performing highly anti-social actions such as murder; or merely that one knowingly exposed oneself unnecessarily to risks of ill-health (perhaps by smoking, heavy drinking, or not exercising (?)). Persons who engage in such courses of action may be said to forfeit their entitlement to health care resources.

It is worth pointing out that, in contrast to a utility-based criterion, the adoption of a desert-based criterion may favour older people at the expense of younger people. This may be the case since the longer a person lives, the greater the opportunities they have had to perform actions such as those referred to in the first two items above. Hence, a desert-based view may redress some of the imbalance which appears to be present in utility-based views, for example.

With respect to the notion of 'negative desert' referred to in the third item above, this could be recruited to ensure that the very young would still have a legitimate claim to health care resources. The specification here also carries the possible merit that those unable to make an economic contribution to a particular society would still be entitled to health care resources, providing they refrained from actions which render them undeserving. Let us turn, now, to consider some of the difficulties raised by proposal of a desert-based criterion.

A first difficulty with the desert-based view is that it appears to be an extremely harsh policy. To focus on the two positive types of criteria referred to above would seem to exclude large numbers of the population, and this simply is not acceptable. The inclusion of considerations relating to negative desert may also appear excessively harsh.

It may be that a person damages their liver by years of heavy drinking. Should such a person be denied access to treatment for the liver damage on the grounds that they brought it upon themselves? Intuitions vary here, but it seems very harsh to judge that the person has forfeited their claim to health care resources. Aside from these points, Professor John Harris ('Heart of the matter: rationing health care', BBC, 27/6/93) raised what seems an extremely difficult problem for the position when it involves appeals to negative desert. The criticism Harris raises is that the fair operation of such a system would require, in effect, the appointment of a 'lifestyle police'. The activities of each citizen would need close and careful monitoring to ensure that each unhealthy action or behaviour is recorded, so that it can be deployed against the citizen should they require health care resources at some future time. Harris thus regards the level of intrusiveness apparently required for the fair implementation of a desert-based view as wholly unacceptable. This seems to constitute a serious criticism to this view: without the inclusion of negative desert it excludes too many citizens; but when negative desert is included, consideration of the practicalities of applying the criterion weigh heavily against its adoption.

Finally, there are two other worries concerning the desert-based view. First, it is not clear how the criterion would apply to new arrivals in a society – be they neonates or people from other countries wishing to settle in that society. If shortly after arrival they require health care resources, how should this situation be coped with? Again, to deny them access to resources sounds brutally harsh. Second, the desert-based view appears to face the same difficulty faced by the other three criteria that have been considered: specifically, how to cope with situations in which equally deserving cases are competing for scarce resources and where both claims cannot be met.

Combining criteria?

Given that each of the four positions considered seems equally problematic, yet each seem to capture something of importance, it may be proposed that the criteria be combined in some way. Such a proposal might recommend that, as a general rule, resources should go to those who need them; but, where this is not possible, other sorts of considerations should be taken into account. So, needing a health care resource marks one as a possible candidate for the receipt of resources, and then other criteria may be brought in to play in the assessment of one's claim. For example, the notions of desert or utility may be said to buttress a claim for resources equally strongly. This approach may help to avoid criticism of the utility-based view to the effect that it unfairly discriminates against older people; and, it may temper the possible bias towards older people in the desert-based view. In spite of difficulties other than that just mentioned which beset the desert-based position, it may well be the case that the last proposal has some merit. This is due to the fact that, as we saw in Chapter 3 earlier, desert does seem to comprise a significant component of our understanding of the concept of justice. More controversially, the same may be claimed of the notion of utility. So, perhaps a feasible criterion of fair distribution can be derived by combining need, utility and desert in some way.

However, a more profitable way forward may be to reconsider relevant moral principles here. In the earlier discussion of justice, Rawls's theory was considered; and it will be recalled that this can be described as a contractarian view. Given the plausibility of the claim that great weight should be accorded to obligations to respect autonomy, it can be suggested that the whole question of how best to allocate resources should be resolved by appeal to what may be termed 'collective autonomy': such decisions should be left to those potentially affected by them. Such a suggestion, in fact, seems to be one for which Rawls's hypothetical 'original position' could be invoked, as discussed in the previous chapter. For example, it may be put to the people in the original position that some access to health care provision should be built in to the state, since it is of course possible that any one of them could be poor and fall ill, or have a condition which requires medical resources (diabetes, asthma, multiple sclerosis, and so on). (For development of such a view, see Green, 1976 and Daniels, 1985.)

Also, such a proposal has the merit of being founded upon respect for the autonomous decisions of persons and, thereby on the principle of respect for autonomy. Persons are being given the opportunity to make informed decisions (decisions based upon awareness of the costs and outcomes of various treatment options) concerning how best to allocate limited resources. It should be emphasized that such a proposal changes the emphasis of questions relating to the distribution of resources. The change is from a consideration of who should be treated, to consideration of which conditions should be treated.

Given acceptance of earlier arguments reporting the importance of autonomy in nursing ethics, it follows that basing a policy of allocation of resources on the principle of respect for autonomy seems well-founded from the moral perspective. Such a proposal has been attempted in practice in Oregon, United States of America (Capuzzi and Garland, 1990; Sipes-Metzler, 1994; Barker, 1995; Beauchamp and Childress, 2009, pp. 268–9). Should its acceptance be recommended in the Unitd Kingdom? Although such a proposal may seem plausible from the moral perspective, there are some serious problems with it, and whether these problems are insurmountable or not I will leave for the reader to judge.

First, in the Oregon Plan, types of health care interventions were prioritized in accordance with 'public values and medical facts' (Capuzzi and Garland, 1990, p. 261; Sipes-Metzler, 1994, p. 305;). These were obtained from a series of public meetings and telephone surveys. All this seems in line with the general, democratic, idea that it is a good thing to base policy upon the views of the electorate. However, grounding public policy on public values may lead to objectionable consequences. For example, given that ageism is widespread in Western cultures, it is not unlikely that programmes of allocation of resources which benefit younger citizens at the expense of older ones would be considered acceptable. Also, in the early days of AIDS awareness in the 1980s, the disease came to be regarded as a problem specific to homosexual males, or to drug users. It is reasonable to judge that widespread prejudice against such groups would militate against the allocation of health care resources to problems associated specifically with them.(See Begg, 2003; the story 'The Gay plague' in NY Magazine, September 1982). This is another kind of concern that can be levelled at attempts to base decisions concerning allocation of health care resources on the autonomy of the relevant constituency.

Second, in contrast to the last worry, it may turn out to be the case that the reports of public values obtained from public meetings and so forth fail to give an accurate representation of the values held by the majority of citizens. This may be because only politically active citizens attend the meetings; or citizens who, say, are employed in health-related occupations (see Benjamin and Curtis, 1992, p. 202).

Third, it may be suggested that the public should not be consulted since they are not experts on health care matters. Hence, this objection queries the legitimacy of the whole approach taken in Oregon and which appears to follow from the emphasis placed on autonomy in the present volume.

Fourth, it may be said that the system of distribution put forward in the Oregon plan is unfair to poor people. This is because rich people will always be able to meet their health needs by purchasing from the private sector. Hence, only poorer citizens will be detrimentally affected by the implementation of the plan.

Responses

When one considers these objections a pattern emerges. The first objection points to a problem in ensuring that the process of consulting the citizens is democratic, in that not all those entitled to express a view may do so; similarly with the second objection. The third objection too tacitly refers to ancient problems with any democratic system. Specifically, these suggest that since members of the electorate are not experts, they are not qualified to make judgements concerning, for example, matters of government or, for that matter, allocation of health care resources.

These objections to democracy were set out persuasively by Plato (in his book *The Republic*). We may describe them as objections concerning the inadequacy of democracy. However, the fact is that the political systems in place in Western cultures are democratic; the selection of governments is performed by the electorate at election times. Surely, if this system of selection of governments is considered acceptable, then it should be considered acceptable when applied to the question of how to distribute health care resources.

The suggestion here, then, is that objections stemming from the claimed inadequacy of the democratic process, or from democracy itself as a political system, are not sufficient to count against the kind of proposal put forward in the Oregon Plan. For, if governments are best chosen by vote, surely systems for the distribution of health care resources are also. This need not mean that every decision is made by referendum. That would not be a practical option. What it could mean, though, is that representatives with health expertise are elected by the electorate to represent their views in matters of health spending.

The fourth objection stated that a system of distribution along the lines of the Oregon Plan is unfair to economically disadvantaged people. This is due to the fact that they alone will bear any harms which result from rationing of resources (at least within the relevant population group). The reason why this charge is legitimate can be seen by reconsideration of points made in our discussion of justice. Suppose two citizens are each covered by a nationwide health plan in which the system of distribution of health care resources is based upon the autonomous wishes of the electorate – call it the UK-Plan. Suppose further that each of our two citizens is in need of an expensive health care intervention which is unlikely to be forthcoming in the terms of the UK-Plan. Such an intervention may be a highly expensive transplant operation, or 24-hour nursing care in the person's own home.

Let us judge that each of these two people is equally needy; however, suppose that one of them is very rich and can afford to pay for the expensive health care intervention, but the other is poor and cannot afford to pay. According to our earlier formulation of the principle of justice in Chapter 3, we are to treat equals equally (and unequals unequally). If the relevant respect in which these two people are equals is that they are equally needy of a specific health care resource, then the poorer person can claim to be the victim of an injustice. For, equals have not been treated equally and, hence, the principle of justice has been violated.

It is important to tread carefully here. As seen earlier, for Rawls, certain properties of individuals are not morally relevant. If it is supposed that the rich person became rich fortuitously – say by virtue of a large inheritance – it may be argued that the two people are indeed equals from the moral perspective. But a morally relevant difference may be claimed to obtain between the rich person and the poor one. For example, this may be said to be the case if the rich person obtained his riches from years of lengthy and hard labour combined with skilful and risky financial judgements.

It is not necessary to comment further here on ways of defending the view that the poorer person is the victim of an injustice, or not, in such circumstances. If one favours Nozick's theory of justice described in the previous chapter, one will be more likely to judge that the poorer person is not the victim of an injustice – merely the victim of misfortune. If one favours a Rawlsian criterion, then one may be much more sympathetic to the claim that the poorer person is indeed the victim of an injustice. The discussion so far has not focused on matters of allocation at the micro-level – at the level of nursing practice. But it is clear that nurses do require an understanding of possible approaches to questions of resource allocation (as noted earlier, perhaps the NMC Code even obliges nurses to have such an understanding).

At the micro-level, nurses, their time and their skills all constitute health care resources. So, a decision taken by a nurse regarding how to manage their time whilst on duty, is a decision concerning resource allocation. As noted, the NMC Code provides a framework of constraints within which nurses have to make decisions. It is not an option to allocate one's time and skills in such a way that one patient is benefited greatly but another is negligently ignored. To plan a regime of care in such a way would be a clear breach of the Code. Hence, nurses' decisions regarding how to allocate their time and skills are constrained by their professional obligations. Given this, a Community Psychiatric Nurse (CPN), say, with a given case-load is obliged to manage his or her time so that the well-being of all patients can be met. This seems to indicate that the criteria for just allocation of nursing time and skills are needs-based: nurses are obliged to try to meet the health care needs of those in their care. This applies to nurses in all contexts. Difficulties arise when nurses find themselves unable to meet such needs, and where this is due to factors beyond their control. For example, it may be the case that in order to meet the needs of their patients, more nurses or more equipment are required. It becomes evident at this point that matters of microallocation are related, eventually, to matters of macroallocation; since, if it is not possible for nurses to meet the needs of their patients given existing resources, decisions have to be made at macro-level concerning questions of health care priorities. Decisions at that level can be influenced by the nurse as a health care professional and as a citizen.

Situations in which nurses are unable to meet the needs of their clients in the sense required by the NMC Code, and in which further resources are not forthcoming, will receive attention in Chapter 6.

Conclusion

This chapter began by discussing moral dilemmas which arise from conflicts between the principles of respect for autonomy, and those of beneficence and non-maleficence. This led into a discussion of the conditions under which paternalistic interventions may be justified, and a discussion of persons who wish to kill or harm themselves. It was, reluctantly, concluded that an autonomy-weighted, principle-based line appears to imply that paternalistic interventions in such instances are extremely hard to justify. An important exemplification of conflict between obligations to respect autonomy and those of justice was then considered; specifically in relation to the allocation of health care resources. After consideration of a number of criteria (utility, rights, needs and desert) a tentative proposal founded on respect for 'collective autonomy' was advanced.

Chapter 5

Care-Based Ethics: A Challenge to the Principle-Based Approach?

The bulk of the present chapter is spent in discussion of a challenge to the principle-based approach from a rival theoretical standpoint – that of a care-based approach to ethics. Since the first edition of this book was published, more work has been done in the field of ethics of care and so it is important to take this into account.

The discussion begins with, and sets aside, a criticism of Beauchamp and Childress's approach which has been advanced by Clouser and Gert, who, it should be stressed, are not themselves advocates of a care-based approach. Once this is done, we examine the nature of the challenge to the principle-based approach presented by care-based ethics. As will be seen, three 'waves' of an ethics of care can be distinguished. Most space is taken up in discussion of the 'first wave' of the ethics of care since this is the most radical and distinctive version. Ultimately, it is argued that the challenge from care-based perspective can be resisted, and a number of problems associated with it are identified. A defence of the principle-based view is attempted. Finally, a position is put forward which we will call a 'principles infused with care' approach. This remains recognizably principle-based, but takes on certain of the legitimate worries which proponents of a care-based approach have with regard to the principle-based line.

First, then, let us turn to Clouser and Gert's well-known critique of Beauchamp and Childress, which as mentioned, is not advanced from a care-based perspective. Our discussion of this will be brief.

Clouser and Gert's critique

This was first presented in 1990 in what has now come to be regarded as a classic paper ('A critique of principlism') and it is mentioned here mainly to make sure readers are aware of it. Clouser and Gert are critical of Beauchamp and Childress in three main ways. These are: (a) that the principles identify a merely arbitrary checklist of moral considerations (1990, p. 220); (b) that the principle-based approach offers no guidance to those faced with moral problems (ibid.); and (c) that when there is conflict between the principles, there is no guidance provided regarding the weighting of the principles (Beauchamp and Childress, 2009, p. 372).

To respond: the second criticism is not really applicable here as, thus far, an approach which does offer some guidance and some rationale for weighting has been offered. And with regard to the first criticism, some of the points made in defence of principle-based approach can be reiterated. Specifically the point that it is plausible to accept that the values captured in the four principles are key anchors of commonsense morality and so the principles provide a well-founded starting point for the analysis of moral problems in health care. In order to respond adequately to such problems it is necessary to have a clear conception of them and as argued previously the principles provide a useful means of doing this. The third criticism has also been dealt with here since an argument has been offered in support of giving greatest weight to the principle of respect for autonomy in the context of health care. Hence, the critique levelled at principle-based approaches by Clouser and Gert can be set aside as we turn to consider the more radical critique presented by an ethics of care.

A care-based approach: the first wave

As mentioned above, since the first edition of this book was published, further work has been done to elaborate an ethics of care, and I find it useful to distinguish 'three waves' of such an approach. Before describing the first version or wave of the ethics of care, it is worth mentioning some contextual details which partly explain the attractiveness of care-based approaches to many within the field of nursing ethics. The view that a focus on caring is something that distinguishes nursing from medicine was widely held at one point (Leininger, 1984; Watson, 1985; Benner and Wrubel, 1989; Fry, 1989). It was thought that whilst caring characterized nursing, curing characterized medicine. Moreover, the idea that these two different kinds of activities should have different approaches to ethical problems proved highly seductive. The view was that an ethics of care is most appropriate for nursing, and an ethics of principles is most suited to medicine. So it is no surprise that many in nursing were drawn to an ethics of care.

The origins of the care-based approach to ethics stem from the work of Carol Gilligan (see her *In a Different Voice, Psychological Theory and Women's Development*, 1982; also Noddings, 1984). Her views developed in part from a reaction to, and rejection of, aspects of the work of the psychologist Laurence Kohlberg (1981). Kohlberg proposed a theory of moral development upon the basis of inviting people to offer their responses to various hypothetical moral problems. He claimed to identify six broad levels of moral thinking from his research data; further, he proposed that these form a hierarchy. At Kohlberg's lowest level of moral thinking, people reason entirely egocentrically; judgements concerning the rightness or wrongness of actions are based solely upon crude consideration of their perceived rewards or punishments for the person concerned. At Kohlberg's highest level of moral reasoning, people deliberate by recruiting universal ethical principles (1981). Actions are morally right insofar as they accord with these principles and result from their employment in moral reasoning.

Gilligan voiced a serious criticism of Kohlberg's claims. She drew attention to the fact that Kohlberg employed only male subjects when conducting the research upon which his conclusions were founded (Gilligan, 1982, p. 18). Gilligan conducted research of her own, this time comparing the way female and male research subjects reason about moral problems. Her conclusions include the claim that female subjects exhibit a 'care-focus' in their moral reasoning, which is much less likely to be present in male subjects (see Gilligan, 1982, 1986). And she went on to distinguish an ethics of care from what she describes an 'ethics of justice'. As we will see, the principle-based approach has the kind of characteristics that Gilligan identifies with an ethics of justice. For now though it is necessary to try to say more about the care-based approach itself as articulated by Gilligan.

In characterizing the care-based view, Gilligan makes use of an example of a moral problem which Kohlberg set his research subjects. In this example, the wife of a man, Heinz, is dying; a chemist has a drug which will save his wife, but Heinz cannot afford to buy it. Kohlberg poses the question, 'Should Heinz steal the drug?' (Gilligan, 1982, p. 26). An 11-year-old male subject, Jake, apparently concludes that Heinz should steal the drug. According to Gilligan, Jake conceives of the dilemma as '[A] conflict between the values of property and life, [and] he uses that logic to justify his choice' (Gilligan, 1982). Gilligan goes on to say that Jake constructs the dilemma 'as an equation and proceeds to work out the solution' (ibid.). Her suggestion is that Jake analyses the moral problem roughly in terms of competing principles, and attaches a weight to these. Since, in Jake's analysis, the life of Heinz's wife counts for more than the wrong done to the chemist by stealing from him, Heinz concludes that stealing the drug is justified.

For Gilligan's purposes, Jake can be seen as a representative of a principle-based view. He approaches the problem coolly, regarding it in the same way that he would regard a problem in mathematics – something to be calculated, and an answer worked out. He employs abstract moral principles such as 'one should not kill' and 'one should not steal' and distils the problem down to a conflict between these. Also, he views the problem as a kind of ahistorical snapshot, again, as one might view an arithmetical problem (see also Alderson, 1992, p. 33 for a similar observation and criticism of the principle-based approach).

Jake's mode of moral reasoning is contrasted with that of another subject, Amy. Gilligan suggests that Amy's construal of the problem is entirely different; she conceives of the problem as a 'narrative of relationships that extends over time' (1982, p. 28). She does not approach the problem by applying abstract moral principles to it. Amy, instead, considers the relationships of the people involved in the problem, and the effects on these relationships of Heinz stealing the drug. In contrast to Jake, Amy manifests some emotional response to the problem, and shows sensitivity to the emotional registers of it (1982, e.g., p. 28). Also, again in contrast to Jake, Amy is reluctant to give a straight answer to Kohlberg's question. Gilligan quotes Amy:

> If he [Heinz] stole the drug, he might save his wife then, but if he did he might have to go to jail, and then his wife might get sicker again, and he couldn't get more of the drug, and it might not be good. So, they should really just talk it out and find some other way to make the money.

And also:

> [Heinz] shouldn't really steal the drug – but his wife shouldn't die either. (1982, p. 28)

Gilligan's proposal that there is a significant difference between the approaches to the problem by Jake and Amy seems a plausible one. Jake's analysis involves distilling and weighing abstract, general principles. Amy, in contrast, seems to focus much more on contextual factors: both the problem and the 'solution' are much less clear-cut for Amy than for Jake. Gilligan, of course, provides other examples in support of her claims to identify a 'different voice' in moral reasoning, but hopefully the example just offered gives an indication of the nature of the difference as Gilligan sees it, between Amy's and Jake's approaches to the problem.

Five claims

In order to try to paint a more detailed picture of the care-based line I find it helpful to ascribe five claims to it, which seem to me to be part of this first wave of the ethics of care and help to signal its distinctiveness. These are: *the uniqueness claim, the caring claim, the emotions claim, the privileged view claim*, and *the Justice Claim*. It should be stressed that these are not terms Gilligan employs herself but terms which I am applying to her approach to try to assess and respond to it.

The uniqueness claim is a claim to the effect that moral problems are unique, they are not the kind of 'repeatable' situations over which generalized principles such as the four principles can usefully be applied (see e.g., 1982, p. 102). This is because in each situation there will be subtle differences such as differing emotional nuances and aspects of the relationship which are relevant to the moral response to them. Amy's reluctance to offer a view about what the right moral response to the Heinz problem stems in part from her appreciation of this. The description of the case is too thin for her to have sense of the emotional nuances involved so how can she express a view since it would be made from a position of ignorance of key factors.

The caring claim is a claim that one's relationships to others are characterized by care (see 1982, pp. 28, 57, 62). One cares about others and wants to help them when they are in need. So, in apparent contrast to the principle-based approach, from a care perspective, one's initial starting point is one of *involvement* with others, not detachment. Thus again Amy's responses manifest sensitivity to the relationships between the parties involved and the desire for them to come together to try to work out a way forward (1982, p. 28). As relationships are characterized by care, when moral problems arise, and since one is involved with those one cares for, one's initial 'reflex' so to speak, is to respond to them. This is in contrast to the justice approach as Gilligan conceives of this since in that, one's 'starting point' is not one of involvement but detachment. One has to be persuaded of the need to respond to moral problems, but in the care approach one simply responds because one is already involved in those problems.

The emotions claim has two aspects to it (1982, p. 28). The first is that emotions are central aspects of the moral life. The second is that they are important guides to action. Thus Amy's response again is sensitive to the emotional registers of the problem, in apparent contrast to Jake. This highlighting of emotions in the moral domain is in stark contrast with other moral traditions in which emotions are regarded as obstacles to development of sound moral responses rather than as facilitators of such appropriate responses.

The privileged view claim (1982, p. 102) is related to the uniqueness claim, and is that since only those in the situation are aware of all the relevant nuances and other subtleties of the situation, they are in a better position than those outside the situation to know how best to respond to it.

The fifth claim – *the justice claim* – is a foundation of this first wave of the ethics of care since Gilligan attempts to develop an ethics that is distinct from an ethics of justice. She goes so far as to claim the two different approaches have differing 'logics' (1982, pp. 73, 30). Certainly, the charge that the principle-based approach relies heavily on justice is a fair one, since, of course, the principle of justice figures as a prominent moral principle within it. Also, it may be said that a reliance on justice is implicit throughout the principle-based approach since, in its application, equals are to be treated equally, and unequals unequally. Moreover, it should be said that the concept of justice is one which has long been at the centre of moral philosophy. Plato, Aristotle and (as seen earlier), more recently Rawls and Nozick have discussed the concept at length. So why might Gilligan and other critics (Okin, 1987; Tronto, 1987, p. 248) be hostile to the view that justice has a central place in morality?

Note that the philosophers listed above as contributors to philo-sophical discussions of justice in morality (Plato, Aristotle etc.) are all male and, further, that a more extensive list would include few female philosophers (see Baier, 1985). Suppose it is suggested that those philosophers who have influenced thought concerning justice developed their initial conception of justice on the basis of their experiences within the family. Such a suggestion is not implausible since Rawls, for example, sets out how the notion of justice derives from interactions within the family (Rawls, 1971, pp. 462–79; Kymlicka, 1990, p. 266). Suppose it is then argued that the fam-ily itself is an unjust social institution. For example, it may be said that the family is maintained by the subjugation of females and that this is manifested, typically, in an unfair division of domestic labour and maintained by economic disenfranchisement of females (see Kymlicka, 1990, chapter 7).

Given acceptance of these two claims, it can then seem plausible to query the legitimacy of the concept of justice which is considered central to moral philosophy. This is so, it may be said, since that con-cept derives from experiences of situations which are themselves unjust (namely, family experiences).

It should be stressed that in this 'first wave' of the care-based approach, a major and mutually exclusive division is asserted between so-called 'justice-based' or principle-based approaches to ethics, on the one hand, and care-based approaches on the other (Alderson, 1990, p. 207). And as noted, Gilligan claims the two different approaches have differing 'logics': 'the logic underlying an ethics of care is a psy-chological logic of relationships, which contrasts with the formal logic of fairness that informs the justice approach' (1982, p. 73). For our purposes, the principle-based view will be regarded as a version of a 'justice-based' approach, and only the more familiar term 'principle-based' will be used henceforth.

The highlighting of these five claims helps to provide a sketch of the care-based view in its first incarnation, but further detail can be added by contrasting it with a principle-based line. This helps to throw the care-based approach into further relief.

Care-based ethics in contrast to principle-based ethics

It can prove extremely difficult to characterize the care-based view, and often it can be illustrated, quite usefully, by contrasting it with a principle-based view (Brabeck, 1983, p. 37). For example, it can be pointed out that the principle-based view emphasizes objectivity and detachment in moral decision-making. This is perhaps most apparent in the principle of justice itself which, as we saw earlier (Chapter 4), is an entirely formal principle bereft of reference to any actual properties or characteristics of individuals. The other principles employed in the principle-based approach can also be said to be abstractions from particular situations or contexts. The principle of non-maleficence, for example, can be regarded as a general principle abstracted from judgements in particular situations that one ought not to inflict harm.

A further example of the emphasis on abstraction and detachment in principle-based approaches can be found in this quote from Singer. He describes a ' Principle of equal consideration of interests' which requires that we 'give equal weight in our moral deliberations to the like interests of all those affected by our action' (1993, p. 21). As with the four principles approach described in the present text, the principle presented by Singer makes no mention of personal relationships that one might be involved in. Thus it seems to imply that the principle should be applied in such a way that even if one's own children or other loved ones are adversely affected by one's action, this fact should not enter into one's moral reasoning behind the action. All that counts from the moral perspective are the interests of those affected by it, the interests of strangers are as important as the interests of those closest to us. This kind of 'detachment' seems a particular feature of principle-based approaches and care-based theorists are correct to query this aspect of them (see also Alderson, 1992, p. 33).

The emphasis upon detachment can also be shown to be present in other responses to moral matters. In the law courts, judges are employed to pass fair punishments upon offenders. The nature of such punishments is not left for those affected by the crime to determine. Also, it is often said that a person is 'too close' or involved with a situation to view it objectively. Perhaps situations where the parents of a child campaign for scarce resources to be allocated to their offspring count here. Even in nursing a nurse may be criticized for being too involved with a patient – for being insufficiently detached from them (Brown, Kitson and McKnight, 1992, p. 39). So, on some views of morality – allegedly including the principle-based view – *the privileged view* claim is implausibly denied. In the care-based view, as we have seen, contextual factors and involvement in situations which are moral problems are each regarded positively.

With respect to notions of involvement in moral problems as opposed to detachment from them (*the privileged view claim*), again the care-based approach places heavy emphasis upon such involvement: the views of the participants in a moral problem have greater, not less, weight than those viewing the problem from a less-involved perspective. And, one's moral obligations, it seems, extend to those one is engaged with in a caring relationship, and for whom one has moral responsibility (see e.g., Gilligan, 1982, p. 19; Tronto, 1987, p. 249; *the caring claim*).

In continuing to attempt to set out the care-based view, use will now be made of three recurring dichotomies which proponents of the view make use of and find especially significant. (The author is indebted to Kymlicka [1990, chapter 7] for much of what follows.) The dichotomies are: public–domestic, objective–subjective, and hierarchy-web. In the discussion, the occurrence of the five claims ascribed to care-based ethics will be signalled as they arise.

Public–domestic

Friedman writes:

> [Morality] is fragmented into a 'division of moral labor' along the lines of gender.... The tasks of governing, regulating social order and managing other 'public' institutions have been monopolised by men as their privileged domain, and the tasks of sustaining privatised personal relationships have been imposed on, or left to, women. The genders have thus been conceived in terms of special and distinctive moral projects. Justice and rights have structured male moral norms, values and virtues, while care and responsiveness have defined female moral norms, values and virtues. (1987, p. 261)

The suggestion here, then, is that a distinction can be made between public institutions and private relationships; the former are described as largely male monopolies, and the latter are left to females. Further, when making moral decisions in public life, it is considered important that these are just, or fair. This, it may be said, is manifested in the (claimed, or aimed for) impartiality of such judgements. Decisions which display favouritism or bias towards a particular group of individuals may be considered unjust since they do not display impartiality. The requirement that politicians reveal their business interests is evidence of this view; as is the obligation on health care professionals not to endorse the products of a particular manufacturer for no reason other than that they are produced by that company.

In marked contrast to the public domain, the domestic domain is conceived to be inhabited mostly by females. Decision-making in this context, it is suggested, is heavily influenced by family relationships (*the caring claim*). The notions of 'care and responsiveness' (Friedman, 1987) are alleged to be the characterizing features of such relationships (*the emotions claim*). The detachment which is an apparent requisite of decision-making in the public domain is supplanted by a (literal) involvement with those affected by the relevant decision. The involvement referred to here is one which is bound up with the notion of caring: one is involved with family members since one cares for them (*the caring claim and the privileged view claim*).

While males in the public domain are concerned with individuals conceived of abstractly as citizens or consumers, females are concerned with individuals defined by their particular characteristics – the properties which are unique to individual persons.

Objective–subjective

We have noted that decision-making in the domestic domain involves phenomena such as feelings, emotions and intuitions (Nicholson, 1983, p. 93) and that these features of moral experience are viewed positively from the care-based perspective. In the theory of knowledge (epistemology), objectivity is associated with truth and knowledge. Truth itself seems importantly bound up with objectivity: if a claim is true, it seems, it is true from all perspectives, so to speak. Further, its truth is open to be discovered. If a knowledge claim is true, it should be possible for another party to verify the truth of that claim. Think especially of knowledge claims made in the sciences here: such claims, it seems, must be open to be verified by scientists other than those who advance the claim. To give an example: imagine that a person claimed to have found a cure for cancer but that it could not be tested by anyone. Would that claim amount to knowledge that the person had a cure for cancer?

These points concerning the notion of objectivity can be taken to support the view that impartiality is a desirable feature of knowledge claims. An enquirer who simply seeks to discover the truth, it may be said, is more likely to succeed than an enquirer who has a vested interest in the success of a particular hypothesis.

The suggestion is that objectivity and impartiality are associated with knowledge and truth. Subjectivity, on the other hand, is associated with lesser notions such as opinion and belief. These may be described as 'lesser' since there is a necessary connection between knowledge and truth – a person can only be said to know that a claim is true, if in fact the claim is true. However, no such necessary connection obtains between opinion and belief, and truth. It may be true that I believe that a claim is true, or that it is my opinion that a claim is true, without its being the case that the claim is in fact true.

Still further, phenomena such as emotions, feelings and intuitions are standardly regarded as subjective phenomena. If moral reasoning is supposed to aim at objectivity, then such data would not be considered relevant to the outcomes of moral decisions. Subjective data such as emotions and feelings are typically thought to impede rational decision-making, and certainly not to enhance it. The distinction between 'objective' and 'subjective' phenomena is intended to distinguish data which are open to view, so to speak, from data which are not. To give an example of the contrast, it may be said that one's height is objective data since, in principle, it can be measured by anyone. By contrast, one's feelings or inner thoughts at a particular time can be described as subjective data since these seem accessible only to the thinking subject.

Proponents of the care-based approach claim that subjective data are essential components of experiences of moral problems, and hence that they should be taken into account in moral decision-making; such data should certainly not be omitted as irrelevant, or as an impediment to moral reasoning (cf. Gilligan, 1982, chapter 5). Alderson says 'Traditions in science and philosophy which mistrust emotion and intuition have to be overcome' (1990, p. 209). Her implication is that moral problems have a subjective element which constitutes legitimate data in moral decision-making – namely, the phenomena of intuition and emotions. Positions in moral philosophy which regard such data as irrelevant are open to strong objection. That is to say, *the caring claim, the emotions claim and the privileged view claim* are highly plausible, and views which do not acknowledge the force of these claims are highly objectionable.

Hierarchy-web

Gilligan describes two ways of conceiving of moral problems, and employs the metaphor of a hierarchy to characterize one of the ways, and the metaphor of a web to characterize the other (1982, pp. 32–3, 48). The hierarchical view is one in which moral problems are surveyed from above, so to speak, looking down on them with 'detached objectivity' (Alderson, 1990, p. 210). Also, in this approach moral principles or rights take their place in a hierarchy of other principles or rights. Allegedly, a view of reasoning about moral problems from this perspective pays little or no attention to emotions experienced – rather like decision-making in the public domain as this was described earlier. Alderson suggests that Ethics Committees tend to adopt such an approach.

In the approach which is characterized by the employment of the web metaphor, people are conceived as being enmeshed in a web of relationships; people are alongside and involved with those experiencing the moral problem and this, in turn, generates a moral problem for them. Anyone towards whom one has responsibilities is, it is claimed, part of this web of relationships (Gilligan, 1982, p. 32); such individuals may include family members, clients, patients and colleagues (*the caring claim*).

Before moving on to try to offer an assessment of the care-based view, it may be worth reiterating some of the main points that have been made. It was noted that Gilligan's work is generally acknowledged as the beginning of the articulation of the care-based view of ethics. She claimed to identify a 'care-focus' in the moral thinking of females. This is held to be distinct from, and superior to, an allegedly male mode of thinking which focuses much more on the weighing of abstract moral principles; the importance of cool, detached deliberation, and the exclusion of emotional responses to moral problems. The latter kind of position closely resembles the principle-based approach. So Gilligan's work aims to identify a 'different voice' (1982) in morality, one in which considerations of involvement in relationships, care and emotional responsiveness are accorded the highest degree of importance.

In an attempt to elaborate the care-based position, three distinctions which care-based theorists exploit have been discussed: public–domestic, objective–subjective and hierarchy-web. These distinctions were exploited to articulate further the care-based view and to distinguish it from the principle-based view. With regard to the public–domestic distinction, this is supposed to indicate that the features of the domestic domain are highly important, and are unduly neglected in moral theorizing. The objective–subjective distinction illustrates the neglect of subjective factors (e.g., emotions) in ethics and indicates the great importance of these in the experience of moral problems. The hierarchy-web metaphor illustrates the differing approaches to ethics represented by principle-based and care-based theorists. Principle-based theorists, it is suggested, view moral problems from 'above' so to speak – from a position of detachment. Care-based theorists, by contrast, hold that the most important perspective on moral problems is that of those involved in the problem, in particular, due to the fact that moral problems arise out of involvement in relations with others.

Hopefully, then, the reader is now clear that the care-based approach involves commitments to the view that moral problems are unique (*the uniqueness claim*); that involvement in certain relations is characterized by care (*the caring claim*); that moral problems are accompanied by the experience of emotions (*the emotions claim*); that those involved in the particular problem have a privileged view of it (*the privileged view claim*); and that an ethics of care is distinct from an ethics of justice because the latter is an inherently dubious concept (*the justice claim*). Let us now turn to look at the position more critically prior to looking in less detail at later versions of the ethics of care.

Criticism of the care-based view (the first wave)

Recall that one of the primary aims of Gilligan's *In a Different Voice* (1982) is to identify a way of understanding, conceiving of and responding to moral problems which is importantly different from that which arises in the principle-based approach. It has been seen in the last section that Gilligan has been successful in achieving this aim. But it needs to be emphasized that the mere identification of a 'different voice' in moral thinking is not by itself sufficient to motivate the wholesale adoption of that voice – by nurses, or by anyone else. Further argument is needed to show that the care-based position is an improvement upon, or superior in some way to the principle-based position.

Thus far, then, Gilligan's work makes, at most, a *descriptive* point: namely, that there is this particular 'care-focused' way of viewing moral problems. But, ethics is a normative enterprise; its concerns are with how people ought to act or reason in relation to moral matters, not simply about how they do, in fact, act or reason about such matters.

What is required, then, is a further argument to show that the care-based view is superior to the principle-based view. In order to arrive at an informed judgement concerning the debate between the two positions, it will prove necessary to set out certain criticisms of the care-based view as it is presented by Gilligan. This task will be undertaken now.

Of course, it may simply be asserted that the care-based is the one which ought to be adopted. But a proponent of the principle-based view might simply make the assertion that, on the contrary, it is the principle-based approach which ought to be adopted. In such a situation it is important that arguments are brought to bear upon the rival views. We have heard some of the worries which opponents (and supporters) of the principle-based view have about that position, and now it is time to consider certain worries which one may entertain about the care-based view.

It should be said at the outset of the criticisms that caring for patients (and others) is indeed a desirable trait in nursing staff and in health care workers generally. However, saying that need not commit oneself to the adoption of care-based ethics. Criticism of the care-based view can usefully focus on the features identified earlier in this chapter and which were deployed in its characterization; namely, the claims of uniqueness, caring, emotions, privileged view and justice. Six objections are made here:

1. The first feature identified was the claim that moral problems are unique, and an objection to this runs as follows. There is a serious problem in emphasizing the uniqueness of moral problems. As Seedhouse points out (1988, p. 94), when one is engaged in moral reasoning – especially as a health care professional – one would like to have some general rules to apply. (Recall the criticisms of 'Act' theories in Chapter 2.) Otherwise, it seems, one could simply be reinventing the wheel on every occasion that one encounters a particular type of moral problem. If one regarded all moral problems as unique, unrepeatable and not, therefore, categorizable into types, then one would not be able to carry over anything learned as a consequence of facing one moral problem, to any other possible moral problem. In short, it seems that generalizations are things we cannot avoid doing if we want to learn from or benefit from our experiences. And further, it seems actually useful – perhaps necessary – to have a set of general moral rules or principles to help is with our deliberations about moral matters. Hence, *the uniqueness claim* seems objectionable.

2. Second, an objection to *the uniqueness claim* related to that just given can be derived from the work of Hare (1981, p. 21; 1952 and Chapter 2 of this text). He draws attention to a logical feature of moral judgements, which is their universalizability. To see how this feature of moral judgements is to be understood, suppose that when faced with a particular moral problem on a particular occasion, one judges that

a certain type of action is the morally correct course of action to take. Hare points out that this commits one to acting in the same way in relevantly similar situations (hence, moral judgements are 'universalizable' to relevantly similar situations). Otherwise, one's moral decision-making is simply arbitrary.

To give an example: Consider that one provides a patient with information concerning the whereabouts of a shop where he or she may purchase cigarettes, even though one would prefer that they did not smoke. Moments later, a patient with the same type of medical condition and generally similar characteristics makes the same request. Given that one judged it right to give the first patient the information she requested, it seems that one ought to give the second the same information – for the same reasons. In fact, Hare's suggestion is that if one judges that in circumstances of a given type (call it type A) that a given course of action is morally correct (call the type of action type T), then one is committed to performing acts of type T in all situations of type A. Insofar as the care-based approach prohibits generalizations from situation to situation or context to context, it seems vulnerable to this objection from Hare, one which stems from consideration of the logic of moral judgements.

3. A third criticism focuses on *the caring claim* and *the privileged view claim*. According to *the caring claim*, caring for others generates moral problems. This, however, can easily be accepted by the principle-based theorist. What is more important in the care-based view is that *the caring claim* is supplemented with *the privileged view claim*: that those involved in moral problems have a more authoritative (privileged) view of them.

It may be said against this position that the care-based view thus encourages what might be termed 'moral bias'. By this it is meant the following. As we have seen, the care-based position places heavy emphasis on the connections between relationships and concern (*the caring claim*). It seems that the domain or extent of one's moral responsibility extends only to those with whom one has a relationship. The term 'relationship' here is of course intended to cover more than simply family relations; let us suppose that it stretches at least to patients, colleagues, close friends, and perhaps further to casual acquaintances. On the face of it, at the very least, from the care-based perspective it would seem that one has stronger moral responsibilities towards those with whom one has relationships than to those individuals who lie outside of these. (This is exploited in the criticism of principles such as Singer's 'Principle of Equal Consideration of Interest described above.) Consider now two examples of moral problems.

In the first example, a parent has a limited budget to use for buying Xmas presents for his or her 10-year-old son. The son badly wants a pair of expensive, designer-label trainers which costs around £150. The parent is aware that this sum of money could go towards a disaster fund to prevent further deaths from a natural disaster which, let us suppose, has recently occurred (e.g., the tsunami in 2004). What should the parent do? It is surely accurate to conclude that from the care-based perspective the parent should give the money to his or her son.

In the second example, suppose that a wife becomes aware that her husband, whom she loves, has committed a terrible crime, perhaps he has murdered a stranger. Suppose, further, that she is aware that her husband may kill again. Should she alert the police and turn her husband in? Again, it seems that from the care-based perspective she should not. She should seek to preserve her relationship with her husband. She has no moral relationship with his potential or actual victims since she does not know them.

Clearly, these are very crude examples of moral problems and they are open to the charge of underdescription. But, it would seem that, in principle, such details could be provided and so objections from the charge of underdescription could be avoided.

The objection being raised, then, is that moral judgements which issue from care-based reasoning exhibit a moral bias in favour of preserving existing relationships; and this may even include situations in which the lives of others are at stake; hence, the charge is that *the privileged view claim* is open to serious objection (see also Tronto, 1987, p. 250).

An obvious way to defend the care-based view from the charge of moral bias is to say that, strictly speaking, people are supposed to have a relationship with all humans – that the web of relationships includes all humans. In fact, Blum asserts 'Gilligan means this web [of relationships] to encompass all human beings and not only one's circle of acquaintances. But how this extension is…to be accomplished is not made clear in her writings…' (Blum, 1988, p. 50; for textual support, see Gilligan, 1982, p. 57). The question of whether all sentient individuals are included in 'the web' also seems pertinent here.

But is this extension of the 'web' a plausible move to make? It involves quite a strained use of the term 'care'. It may be said of me that I care for persons whom I am acquainted with and related to. It may be said of a nurse that he cares for those to whom he has a professional responsibility. But to say that a person cares for, say, a stranger in another part of the world – a part perhaps that the person has never heard of and has no conception of – seems a very odd sense of 'care' to rely upon. To say that a person Smith cares for Jones or any other person, seems to involve, at the very least, the claim that this is the result of some actual thought about Jones by Smith; this is implausibly denied in the response under discussion.

Also, recall that part of the appeal of the care-based approach stemmed from considerations arising from involvement in a caring relationship with a person. Again, this militates against applying the concept of care to situations in which persons do not even know of each other's existence. Hence, this third criticism of the care-based view seems a powerful one.

4. A fourth objection again focuses on *the privileged view claim*, and draws upon that derived from Hare and discussed in the second criticism just offered. Apart from the apparent logical properties or features of moral judgements, it surely is incumbent upon nursing staff not to be morally arbitrary in their moral decision-making. This seems a distinct possibility if the sole constraints on moral decision-making are those which issue from the care-based perspective (specifically that one's moral judgements are informed solely by considerations of care). It is, of course, required of nursing staff that they be accountable. As we heard in our discussion of the principle-based view, this amounts to offering explanations of one's decisions and actions. Within the parameters of health care practice, professional considerations constrain moral theorizing. However, it seems that the sole explanation one can offer in support of moral decisions from the care-based view is that one's motives were sound ones – they were motivated by care and concern. But this is not enough. Care is important, but these considerations do not exhaust those relevant to moral decision-making in nursing practice.

Further, it is evident that more justification is required for moral actions than the mere fact that they were undertaken out of considerations of care. To see this, consider that a parent, out of care for their children, insists that they have a cold shower at 5.00 a.m. each morning; or that they go without food one day a week. When pressed for reasons, the parent says that their actions are sincerely motivated by care for their offspring. In the health care context, suppose that a patient is allowed to die against his or her wishes. Suppose, further, that the patient's death results from a nurse intentionally omitting to resuscitate him or her. (For discussion of such a case, see Curtin and Flaherty, 1982, p. 294.) The actions of the nurse may well be motivated by considerations of care – perhaps he or she thought the degree of suffering being endured by the patient too great – but the further question of whether their actions are morally justified is pressing.

5. A fifth criticism to be offered here is that the care-based line has within it an importantly damaging logical inconsistency (Blum, 1988, pp. 57, 62). The charge of logical inconsistency is quite a straightforward one. Recall that in the care-based approach it is regarded as essential to consider particular moral problems as unique, context-based, non-repeatable situations. Approaches, which seek to make generalizations, or to make judgements based upon principles supposedly applicable to types of situations, are deemed inappropriate – due to *the uniqueness claim*. Put another way, moral claims which are supposed to carry universal applicability are ruled out on the care-based line. But, it is apparently claimed at the same time that the care-based approach itself is one which is applicable across a great many, perhaps all, moral problems. The difficulty here is one common to theses which seek to exclude general claims. Evidently, in seeking to rule out general claims one makes a general claim – a claim applicable to a broad class of cases. It may be said that this logical difficulty can be accepted. But even if this is true, it seems to be being claimed that the care-based view is in fact a view which makes a general – dare one say universal – claim for its applicability. (I am indebted to Blum, 1988, here.)

6. With regard to the justice claim, our response to this can also be taken to apply to the objection to the principle-based approach regarding its 'unjust concept of justice' (see above Okin, 1987; Tronto, 1987). It can be agreed from the outset that most of the standard philosophical authorities on theories of justice are males. Further, it should be agreed that, presumably, most of these authorities lived in families, and perhaps it is the case that the domestic arrangements in these families reflected broader social prejudices which included sexism against females.

In some respects this is a peculiar criticism. Recall in our discussion of Gilligan's claims that it was pointed out that, at most, she provides descriptive points; and that further argument is required to compel us to adopt the way of thinking about ethics which is found in the 'different voice'. A directly parallel response can be made here. It can be accepted that those philosophers who have most influenced philosophical thought on justice were brought up in an unjust social institution – the family; and perhaps even in an unjust society. This seems especially true of Plato and Aristotle. In ancient Athens, females and 'slaves' were apparently denied any say in the affairs of the state.

However, this is again, a descriptive point. It does not show the thinking of those philosophers about justice to be fatally flawed. It could even be suggested that the very injustice of the social arrangements which surrounded them prompted them to think carefully about what justice consists in.

Further, it should be said that the formal definition of justice quoted from Beauchamp and Childress, and drawn from Aristotle, which we considered above, in fact helps to show just why sexism is unjust. In sexist societies or social institutions, individuals are discriminated against upon the basis of characteristics which are not relevant from the moral perspective – namely, their sex, the colour of their eyes, how tall they are, and so on. So again, the principle-based view can be defended against the present objection.

The above criticisms have mentioned three of the four main aspects of the care-based approach, but no mention has been made of *the emotions claim*. As noted, this can be understood in two ways, one of which is plausible and will be accepted here, and the other of which is not plausible and will be rejected. The plausible interpretation of the claim is that emotions are an important feature of moral experience. Of course one can be moved by the plight of others, and such emotional responses seem important, especially if they drive us to actually try to do something to relieve the plight of others, for example where this involves terrible suffering or other forms of hardship. This seems an important aspect of moral experience. The implausible interpretation of this claim is that emotions are a reliable guide to moral responses. In the heat of the moment one's emotional response might be to strike someone who has done a great wrong to one, or one's family. This would be an emotional response of course. But it does not follow that it is the morally right response. This is partly why sentencing of criminals is left to judges in the law courts rather than to the victims of crime or their relatives. If the care-based approach involves this stronger interpretation of the emotions claim then it is not plausible for the reason just offered.

With reference to the three dichotomies mentioned above, some criticisms of a principle-based approach implied by these also need to be addressed before we can move on. The dichotomies are those between the public and the domestic domain, between objectivity and subjectivity, and between the metaphors of hierarchy and web.

The public–domestic dichotomy is exploited to try to show that there are two moralities which correspond to the two spheres – the public and the domestic. And, the implication is that the principle-based approach may be appropriate in the public domain but is not in the domestic. Further, as we saw, this dichotomy is articulated in terms of gender too.

Interestingly, though, nursing occupies a position somewhere between the public and the domestic spheres. This is because of the kinds of considerations rehearsed in Chapter 1 above. Although a hospital is a public place, within it patients dress in ways which are not typical of the public domain. They wear night clothes, often. And the relationships between patients and nurses are not like those which obtain in more formal public settings. So the nursing context is not quite like the public domain, nor is it quite like the domestic domain of course, since it is inhabited largely by strangers. So even if one is persuaded that there is this public–domestic dichotomy, nothing really follows from that as far as acceptance or rejection of the principle-based approach is concerned. For reasons given in our discussion of justice, a nurse has to think about matters of fairness when allocating her own time and other health care resources. Yet of course, care is also a feature of the nursing role. But to note this is, again, not yet to show the principle-based approach to be fundamentally flawed or inappropriate for the nursing context.

The objective–subjective dichotomy raises differences in emphasis between the care-based and principle-based views. A supposed merit of the care-based position is that so-called subjective phenomena are taken into account in moral decision-making. The implicit objection is that the principle-based approach devalues such phenomena or regards them as impairments to moral decision-making.

But the principle-based line can be applied in such a way as to acknowledge the importance of subjective phenomena such as emotions. As was recognized above, very frequently moral problems are accompanied by experiences of psychological distress. It is important to discuss the way it feels to be engaged in a moral problem. This can be of great educational benefit in addition to helping nurses learn from their experiences of moral problems in practice. So, it cannot be said that a principle-based approach must necessarily exclude all reference to subjective phenomena.

Perhaps it will be said that the fundamental difference between the two approaches is the weight attached to subjective phenomena. It is accurate to state that in the principle-based line great emphasis is attached to the employment of reason and informed debate about moral problems. These are associated with objective enquiry. Reasons for holding a position are requested, examined, defended and either retained or rejected. This kind of procedure for evaluating between incompatible claims is common (essential?) to all academic disciplines. Proponents of the principle-based view argue that these types of constraints on theorizing are extremely valuable. One is usually better equipped to assess the force of a case when one has heard the arguments for and against it.

It seems that proponents of the care-based line, in its early form at least, wish to pit against this picture of rational debate, a position in which there are no constraints in disputes about moral matters. What matters most, it seems to be said, is what one feels one should do, irrespective of rational assessment. But if reason is not a constraint in moral debate, then there can be no moral arguments and each position is as legitimate as any other. This is a view known as moral subjectivism. Some find this position attractive, but it is easily shown to be vulnerable to extremely serious objections (see especially, Midgeley, 1991).

To give a brief indication of why moral subjectivism may be thought objectionable, recall that for its proponents any moral view is as legitimate as any other. Suppose, now, one person claims it morally right to torture children for sexual gratification, and another person disagrees. For the moral subjectivist, there is no further discussion which can take place here: matters of right and wrong are simply matters of individual judgement. There are more technical and adequate objections to the position than that those just offered (Edwards, 1990; Midgeley, 1991). But, hopefully, the reader can see the danger in moral subjectivism and in positions which deny a role for reason in moral debate. The suggestion being that this is a danger into which the first articulation of the care-based position seems to fall.

It can be repeated again that a position which denies a role for reason in moral debate is not really one which accountable professionals can adopt and at the same time hope to meet their professional obligations. These require nurses to offer reasons in support of their decisions and not simply to base their decisions entirely on emotional grounds – though, it needs to be stressed, the importance of such elements of experience of moral problems is not being downplayed.

With respect to the hierarchy-web dichotomy, the claim here was that in the care-based approach moral problems arise among persons who are engaged in a 'web' of social relations. In contrast, the principle-based approach was said to be hierarchical in at least two ways: first, in that those making moral decisions were claimed to 'look down' upon those involved in the relevant moral problem; and, second, in that one or other moral principle is accorded a 'higher' position in the approach than other considerations.

Consider the first of these charges. In response it can be pointed out that persons employing the principle-based approach in moral decision-making need not be conceived of as looking down upon the persons involved in the moral problem. For example, you may be a nurse sympathetic to the principle-based approach and you may be involved in a moral problem – either during the course of your professional duty or in some other part of your life. Evidently, people who have moral decisions to make are also engaged in social relationships (of course, these include professional relationships too). So, a person who 'looks down' upon individuals involved in a moral problem is perhaps forgetting that they too are involved in the problem and so cannot consider themselves detached from it.

With regard to the second charge, it should be conceded that in the principle-based approach as it has been set out here, it has been argued that the principle of respect for autonomy should be considered as the most weighty principle. But, this position is not one randomly plucked out of the air, but rather one which has been motivated by argument. Hence, it would seem to this author that the second charge does not need further response.

Before moving on, it may be wise to reiterate some of the reasons which are being taken here to lead to acceptance of a principle-based view (though one in which certain subjective phenomena are recognized as legitimate) and rejection of a care-based view of the kind set out by Gilligan.

Attempts to show one approach to ethics to be more adequate than another raise quite serious methodological difficulties. But one way to assess rival approaches is to test them for internal consistency. Consistency, it can be said, is a constraint on any approach put forward in any subject matter. It should be expected of any view that it does not contradict itself, and this can be described as a condition of adequacy on any approach. However, as we saw earlier, the care-based approach seems not to meet this condition of adequacy. By contrast the principle-based line seems not to contain any internal contradiction.

A second constraint, or condition of adequacy to which any approach is subject is that deriving from considerations of meaning: does the approach make sense? It can reasonably be proposed that both the approaches under consideration here satisfy this second condition of adequacy.

These last two conditions are uncontroversially applicable to all moral theories and approaches to health care ethics. However, it seems plausible that the two constraints just described do not go far enough in terms of their applicability to nursing ethics. The reason is that any approach to nursing ethics must be compatible with the conditions which constrain professional practice (Edwards, 2006). Hence, it would count against a proposed approach if it was not compatible with the professional obligations of nursing staff. It seems to me that the care-based view suffers from such an inadequacy. The reasons are those already mentioned. The care-based view appears to lead to moral subjectivism, and this is incompatible with the professional obligations which bind nurses. The clauses of the NMC Code oblige nurses to act in certain types of ways – ways which seem easily characterized by the use of moral principles. Also, the care-based approach seems to encourage a case-by-case approach to nursing ethics. Again, as seen earlier, it is not clear that this is either possible or helpful. And, finally, for by-now familiar reasons, the care-based approach appears not to require further justification for moral decisions other than that they were motivated by care. It was argued above that this is not sufficient justification for actions undertaken by accountable professionals.

In summary, then, the care-based approach can be subjected to at least the above criticisms, most of which seem powerful ones. Before we can begin to articulate a preferred position, further tasks need to be accomplished. We need to describe the second and third waves of the ethics of care. The discussion of second and third waves can be done much more briefly than the discussion of the first wave. This is because, as we will see, these later versions of an ethics of care share much more in common with the principle-based approach.

The second wave

We saw that Gilligan exploits a distinction between care and justice, implying that these are mutually exclusive. What marks the second wave of care ethics is that a key place is made for justice (Tronto, 1993; see also Card, 1990; van Hooft, 1995; Bowden, 1997). The criticisms given above against Gilligan's version of an ethics of care illustrate that an approach to ethics which jettisons commitment to justice, although radical, is unlikely to be plausible. Hence, Tronto accepts that a theory of justice must have a fundamental place in an ethics of care because this ' is necessary to discern among more and less urgent needs' (1993, p. 138; also Card, 1990). It is this inclusion of justice which marks a crucially different kind of ethics of care than is present in the first wave.

Whilst rejecting the care/justice dichotomy, Tronto sets up a different one to try to articulate an ethics of care as distinct from other approaches, such as a principle-based approach. In order to do this, she exploits one of the themes from the first wave, which is that of responsibility in relationships with others – something captured above in *the caring claim*. Thus Tronto distinguishes between obligation-based and responsibility-based approaches in morality. A principle-based approach to ethics would be categorized as an obligation-based approach according to Tronto's distinction. This is because, as we saw, the principles are understood to refer to moral obligations and to capture these. As explained above, the principle of respect for autonomy refers to obligations to respect autonomy, the principle of beneficence refers to obligations to be beneficent, and so on.

Also the so-called impartial 'moral point of view' which is a feature of other approaches to ethics is not accepted by Tronto. Again, Singer's Principle of Equal Consideration of Interests can serve as an example of a principle which may be thought to presuppose an impartial moral point of view, from which responses to moral problems are calculated. So too would the principle-based approach, together with the utilitarian and deontological theories we considered in Chapter 2. The reason is that, as Tronto sees these, they begin from an initial position of non-involvement. Such positions can be seen in terms of the 'hierarchy-web' dichotomy which is a feature of Gilligan's analysis. Tronto follows Gilligan in this respect.

In contrast to such approaches, it is said that as human beings our predicament is one of involvement, not the detachment 'valorised' in the 'moral point of view' perspective (i.e., the principle-based, utilitarian and deontological approaches etc.).

Also, as noted traditional theories are 'obligation-based', but the ethics of care is 'responsibility-based' (see also Gilligan, 1982, pp. 73, 74). The contrast that Tronto is pointing to here can be illustrated as follows. In obligation-based approaches, as Tronto see these, when one becomes aware of the plight of another one considers what obligations, if any, one has to help that person. Upon the basis of such consideration, one decides whether or not one is under an obligation to respond. There is a presumption of separation between moral agents; and obligations to others need to be justified, they are not presumed.

By contrast, in a responsibility-based ethic of care, the presumption is, instead, one in which there is a pre-existing moral relationship or 'connection' between people. So obligations are presumed and are not in need of justification.

In addition to the emphasis on responsibility which we have just described, Tronto claims that an ethics of care is a practice: 'Care is...best thought of as a practice' (1993, p. 108), not as an 'emotion' or as a 'principle'. '[Care] involves both thought and action, that thought and action are interrelated, and...are directed to some end' (1993, p. 108; also van Hooft, 1995). An ethics of care involves 'a "habit of mind" to care' (ibid., p. 127). So to care is not just to be emotionally moved by the plight of others, but to act to help them.

As part of this practice, Tronto posits 'Four ethical elements of care' (1993, p. 127). These are: (a) attentiveness, which is the 'recognition of need' (p. 127); (b) Responsibility, she intends this in the sense of 'taking care of' (p. 131), such that there is a presupposition of responding and not of needing persuasion that there is an obligation to help others; (c) Competence, this is to signify that the caring must be competently executed (p. 133); (d) Responsiveness (p. 134), this seems to concern not so much the care giver as the care receiver as Tronto writes of 'the responsiveness of the care receiver to the care' (p. 134). However, the point is developed by reminding us of the essential vulnerability of humans: 'To be in a situation where one needs care is to be in a position of some vulnerability' (1993, p. 134). (See also Noddings, 1984 on the part of the 'cared-for' in an ethics of care.)

Thus one can see that this second version of the ethics of care is a definite departure from the first wave. The inclusion of a role for considerations of justice is plainly crucial and distinctive. This marks out the second wave of the ethics of care from the first wave. Also, in setting out the contrast between the ethics of care and the principle-based approach, as seen, Tronto makes use of the distinction between responsibility-based approaches (within which an ethics of care lies) and obligation-based approaches (within which the principle-based approach is said to lie). Let us move on, then, to look more critically at Tronto's approach.

Comment and criticism

In this renewed version of an ethics of care, as we have noted, the key feature of it is the attempt to incorporate a role for the idea of justice.

This ensures that one distributes goods fairly, and not in a biased way. So it marks a substantial departure from the version championed by Gilligan. Also, *the caring claim* is retained and filled out. We are told that caring is a practice, a way of responding habitually to others in caring ways. No commitments are evident to *the uniqueness claim* or to the stronger interpretation of *the emotions claim*. Thus it avoids objections stemming from adherence to these.

Articulation of the sense in which what remains is still an ethics of care focuses on the claims made above. These are:

- a rejection of the 'moral point of view' allegedly a feature of more traditional approaches;

- an emphasis on responsibility as opposed to obligation;

- the idea of care as a practice;

- the four ethical elements of care: attentiveness, responsibility, competence, and responsiveness.

In the responses to these four aspects to be given now, it will be shown that there is no fundamental incompatibility between this version of an ethics of care and the kind of principle-based approach developed here (or even that developed by Beauchamp and Childress themselves) when applied to nursing ethics.

To see this, consider the first of the bulleted items above. This can be responded to by pointing out that if the idea of the moral point of view is of a wholly neutral vantage point from which one devises responses to moral problems, then there is no commitment to such a position in the principle-based approach. The approach was devised with health care professionals in mind to try to help them respond ethically to problems in health care practice. So even if more traditional theories presuppose a hypothetical, abstract 'moral point of view' there is no such commitment in the principle-based approach. One can endorse a principle-based approach and at the same time recognize that we are all situated in some context or other – we are related to others in various ways as parents, colleagues, friends, nurses, and so on. So one can recognize the 'situated' nature of each of us and at the same time maintain that as 'situated' people our responses to moral problems can be usefully informed by the four principles.

With regard to the second point, as this is a book on *nursing ethics* it is sufficient simply to point out that responsibility to others is an essential part of the nurse's role. Hence, the 'starting point' of involvement which this emphasis on responsibility to others signals is already present in the nursing context. Moreover, again I see no conflict with adherence to a principle-based approach in recognizing this. Knowing that one is responsible for the care of others, one wants to respond to the ethical dimension of that relationship. The principles again, at least, provide a structure to enable one to work out how best to enact that responsibility.

In response to the proposal that an ethics of care is neither a principle nor an emotion, but a practice, again there might not be much to object to about this. The idea that nursing itself is a practice has received much attention in recent years (Wainwright (1997), Sellman (2000)) and conceivably this kind of idea could be developed in support of such a view. But in terms of our specific agenda here, there is no incompatibility between viewing care as a practice if it involves 'thought and action...directed to some end' as Tronto puts it (1993, p. 108). This is because the 'end' referred to could, of course, be that of fostering and respecting the autonomy of patients, or of trying to benefit them or treat them fairly and so on.

With regard to the fourth bullet point and the four ethical elements of care, again I see nothing that conflicts with a principle-based approach. The idea of attentiveness was discussed, although in different language, in Chapter 1. There we highlighted the importance of moral perception and sensitivity. As discussed in that chapter, it is important that nurses cultivate their moral perception so they can recognize and respond to ethical dimensions of their practice. The example (Chapter 1 above) of the uncomfortable patient in the bed whose discomfort was spotted by one (attentive) nurse and missed by her colleague was given to illustrate the importance of this. For present purposes it is plain there is no incompatibility between emphasizing the importance of this capacity and a principle-based approach. The element of responsibility has already been dealt with above. The importance of competence is plain and there is nothing to dispute there: of course if one cares for others, the care one gives should be done competently. The fourth element, responsiveness, emphasizes the vulnerability of those being cared for. This does not present a problem for principle-based approaches either. The reason is that the vulnerability of patients – indeed, of human beings per se – is obvious. We are all vulnerable to illnesses, accidents and misfortunes. But it need not follow from this that the kinds of obligations captured in the principles need to be underplayed. Given that one is vulnerable, surely it remains important that one's autonomy is cultivated and one's decisions respected, that one is treated fairly, that others consider one's best interests, and so on.

Evidently, then, this second wave of the ethics of care presents no serious challenge to the principle-based view, as far as I can see anyway. The recognition of the indispensability of some principle of justice renders this second wave more plausible than the first wave. But in doing so, it does not present any significant challenges to a principle-based ethics. As we will now see, the same is true of the third wave.

The third wave

A third wave, following Little and Verkerk, sees an ethics of care as a 'moral orientation' (Little, 1998, p. 191; Verkerk, 2001). As Gastmans expresses it;

> I claim that a care ethic stands on its own...as a 'moral perspective or orientation' from which ethical theorizing can take place. This will mean that care ethics is more a stance from which we can theorize ethically rather than a full-blown ethical theory in itself. (2006, p. 146)

This observation comes towards the close of a very clear chapter on the ethics of care. More to the point for our purposes, this quote itself, as I understand it, indicates no incompatibility between an ethics of care and a principle-based approach (also Nortvedt, 1996). This is because one can take the very formulation of the principles as stemming from an attitude of care. Thus because one is concerned about – cares about – the plight of those involved in health care, as patients, potential patients, or carers, and so on, one tries to respond to their plight in the best way possible. So if the formulation of the four principles is seen in that way it too can be seen as stemming from a 'moral perspective or orientation' and to be a product of subsequent ethical theorizing.

Thus, due to the possession of moral awareness and perception one recognizes problems as moral ones, and wrestles with them because one cares about the plight of others and is driven by a responsibility to try to respond to them. This can be cultivated in moral education by developing the moral perception, sensibility and imagination of others. As Tronto's account brings out, it is not enough simply to have well developed faculties of moral awareness and perception. These make it possible for one to notice moral aspects of experience, but say nothing about *responding to* those aspects. As is emphasized in Tronto's version, care is manifested by the fact that one responds to a situation as opposed to simply perceiving it and not responding. Thus recall again our example of Mrs Jones in Chapter 1. Suppose Freda, having noticed Mrs Jones' discomfort, simply walks past her. This might display excellent moral perception but is plainly a failure to care for Mrs Jones. Care highlights the importance of actually responding to moral perceptions, to try to do something about them if needed.

Hopefully, then, it is clear at least what later versions of the ethics of care are highlighting. They serve to remind us that to be moral is to do more than simply notice moral problems, it is to respond to them. For some people at least, it is due to this caring sensibility that they are led into health care work. They recognize the suffering of others as a moral dimension of human experience, and want to try to respond to it.

As mentioned, however, the second and third versions of ethics of care do not seem to me to present a serious challenge to a principle-based approach. There is no reason why the points about responsiveness, for example, need be denied by anyone sympathetic to a principle-based approach. It is perfectly compatible with using the principles to structure one's moral responses to the problems one's moral perception has brought to one's attention. Thus by virtue of moral awareness and perception we become aware of the moral dimension of situations, and an orientation to care prompts us to respond to those situations. The four principles can be used to structure those responses. Hence, responses should be structured in terms of respecting autonomy, promoting well being, not harming and being fair.

To recap our discussion of an ethics of care then. We began by outlining Gilligan's attempt to devise an ethics of care which is distinct from an ethics of justice. As seen, this ran into several problems. But some aspects of the ethics of care were noted as important; in particular, the recognition of the importance of emotions in the moral domain, the importance of relationships, and of viewing moral problems as narratives as opposed to 'snap shots'. We also noted the importance of the critique of justice-based approaches to the effect that they 'privilege' detachment over involvement, in spite of the fact that, ultimately, this critique was not found to be compelling. The second and third waves of an ethics of care although evidently more plausible than the first wave, could not be found sufficiently distinct from a principle-based approach. Hence the position arrived at is one in which the general claim advanced in the third wave of the ethics of care is endorsed, but which need not lead us to abandon principle-based ethics. Thus one notices moral problems because one cares about others, and once one has noticed them, the principles provide at least a starting point in that they enable the person to 'frame' the problem and so try to formulate a response to it. In terms of nursing ethics, the nurse seems inevitably led to consider values captured in the principles, autonomy, beneficence, non-maleficence and justice. These are, as it were, 'overlaid' upon a bedrock of care, or in the terms used in Chapter 1 above, a bedrock of moral awareness and perception. So there is no incompatibility between care and respect for autonomy, nor between care and justice.

In the final section in this chapter, we will try to say a bit more about the nature of the kind of principle-based approach which is being presented here. As can be seen, this is described as a 'principles infused with care' approach (or more simply, but less accurately, a 'principles plus care' approach, Edwards, 2007).

'Principles infused with care' approach

As mentioned previously, attempts in ethics to defend one particular approach in preference to another present considerable problems of method. For example, what kinds of considerations could be relevant? In other disciplines if there is a dispute between two rival theories a test situation is devised and the theories evaluated in the light of the test situation. If Smith claims that water freezes at 0 degrees C but Jones claims that water freezes at 2 degrees C, their respective claims can be put to the test. But it is not quite so easy to devise a test situation to prove which of two rival approaches to ethics is most superior. How could approaches to ethics be subjected to tests of the kind to which the claim that 'water freezes at 2 degrees C' can be? Certainly discussion of the application of the rival approaches to hypothetical or actual examples of moral problems can play an important role in such a process of evaluation. Having drawn attention to this methodological worry, it should be said that some progress can be made. We have seen that the first care-based view suffers from a number of serious problems.

To try to illustrate how the kind of principle-based approach being defended here would apply in practice, consider this example. It was developed originally in the first edition as a response to the criticism that the principle-based approach is 'callous and uncaring' and places greatest emphasis upon respecting autonomy in the sense of 'non-interference' with the wishes of others (Alderson, 1992, p. 33).

These are the kinds of moral failings which, of course, care-based approaches to ethics are intended to address, and in arguing above that such approaches are either dubiously coherent (first wave) or compatible with a principle-based approach (second and third waves), it will be useful to explain further how one can adopt a principle-based approach to ethics and yet remain caring.

The case example is as follows. It concerns the moral problems raised by caring for patients who are in need of pressure-area care. Specifically, the difficult moral problem faced when a patient who, in the nurse's considered view is in urgent need of pressure-area care, competently refuses such care. Suppose two nurses – call them nurse A and nurse B – have been introduced to the rudiments of the principle-based approach to nursing ethics and are familiar with difficulties concerning the relationship between respect for autonomy and paternalism.

Nurse A simply states that as far as he is concerned, if a patient refuses pressure-area care, knowing the consequences of such a refusal, then the patient's wish should be respected – as is required, perhaps, by the obligation to respect their autonomy.

Nurse B's approach seems to differ, in what seems to me to be an important way. Suppose this nurse says that in such a situation he would not take the patient's refusal at face value, so to speak. He (nurse B) would try to enter into a dialogue with the patient, asking whether there was anything that he, the patient, was concerned about. Having given the patient the opportunity to mention anything that was of concern to him, the nurse would ask the patient again if his pressure-area care could be carried out. Suppose Nurse B adds that if the patient still refuses, then the obligation to respect their autonomy should be respected.

As a patient, it occurs to me that I would prefer to be in the care of nurse B than nurse A. It does, indeed, sound as though A's implementation of the principle-based approach has 'a chilly, uncaring emphasis on respect as non-interference' (Alderson, 1992, p. 33). But, it would seem wholly wrong to say this of nurse B's approach to the situation. In nurse B's approach his obligations to the patient of beneficence and respect for autonomy are considered in a way which is *infused with care*. Even though, ultimately, nurse B decides to respect the competent, autonomous wish of the patient to forgo his pressure-area care, this decision is made from considerations informed by the principle-based approach and as a result of caring about the patient. Ultimate weight is carried by principle-based considerations, though care-based considerations are not neglected or seen as irrelevant (see also Blum, 1988, p. 55).

So, in response to the charge that the principle-based approach fosters a callous and uncaring attitude among nursing staff, it can be pointed out that the approach can be applied in a manner which is infused with care, or less technically, manifests a caring disposition towards patients (and, of course, colleagues). To try to say a bit more about what being 'infused with care' amounts to the work of one of the early contributors to work on the ethics of care can be turned to, Nel Noddings (1984). With specific reference to the question of how the term 'care' is to be understood, Noddings proposes that, in her view, caring involves a 'displacement of interest from my own reality to the reality of the other' (1984, p. 14). She asserts:

> Apprehending the other's reality, feeling what he feels as nearly as possible, is the essential part of caring from the view of the one-caring. (1984, p. 16)

And:

> Caring involves stepping out of one's own personal frame of reference into the other's. When we care, we consider the other's point of view, [and]...his objective needs. (1984, p. 24)

On this view, from the perspective of the carer, caring necessarily involves the attempt to see things from the position of the person cared-for 'as nearly as possible', and also considering and respecting the 'objective needs' of the cared-for. There are some difficulties with Noddings's claims, but on a sympathetic reading they are plausible and helpful. They also amount to a strategy which can be deployed to try to develop what we called, following Scott (1995) and others, 'moral imagination' in Chapter 1.

The idea is that in caring for another, it is helpful to try to place oneself as closely as possible in the position of the person cared for, and to try to assess the situation from their point of view. As Noddings is aware, literally speaking, it is not possible to do this since obviously one cannot actually step inside another person's head and see the world exactly as they see it; and it is often very difficult to judge what a person's 'objective needs' might be. But, when one is engaged in caring for another it seems necessary to at least consider what the best interests of the person cared for may be, as far as one is able to judge. Of course what the patient says they need is an important resource to aid such assessments. And when patients are unable to speak, we know there are some needs common to all humans, those for food, water, air, comfort, freedom from unwanted pain etc. Further, the carer is obliged to act upon their assessment of a patient's 'objective needs'.

On such a view, then, caring for unconscious patients amounts to considering the person's plight as much as possible from the perspective of the unconscious person, and acting upon what are judged to be the best interests of the person. With regard to conscious patients, an obvious and sensible way to try to determine just what the interests of a patient are, is to ask them. One might do this simply by spelling out the options available to them in terms which the patient can make sense of. This is simply to respect obligations of autonomy. Of course, if the patient is unconscious, one needs to consider their perspective on their behalf without the benefit of their own views.

Given this crude but hopefully plausible proposal on just what caring might be thought to include let us return to the saga of nurse A and nurse B and the moral problem of how to care for the patient in need of pressure-area care but who is refusing it. It was suggested above that nurse B's implementation of the principle-based approach is infused with care: relevant moral principles are applied but in a caring manner. By contrast, nurse A's application of the principles did appear to display the chilly, uncaring aspect which Alderson (1992, p. 33) detects in principle-based approaches.

It should now be possible to try to fill out just what is meant by the claim that the principle-based approach can be implemented in a way which is infused with considerations of care. In the nurse A/nurse B example, nurse A simply informs the patient that the patient is in need of pressure-area treatment at that time, and asks if this is acceptable to him or her. This, it may be said, amounts to respecting the autonomy of the patient. Since the patient refuses the treatment, nurse A leaves him alone – again, a response ostensibly grounded in respect for autonomy. No caring response is manifested by nurse A.

Nurse B handles the situation differently. Although he recognizes and is ultimately prepared to respond to obligations to respect autonomy, he considers the interests of the patient as he sees them. Recalling Noddings's expression 'as nearly as possible', it is evident that if the patient's pressure areas are neglected, then tissue damage will inevitably occur. So, the patient's response at least jars with what would appear to be his or her best interests; that is, even when an attempt is made to consider what these may be from the perspective of the patient. This mismatch between the nurse's judgement of what is in the patient's best interests, and the patient's own refusal of the pressure-area care, prompts nurse B to take the interaction into another phase. In trying to view the situation as much as possible from the perspective of the patient, he invites the patient to discuss the fears, emotions and reasons behind the refusal of treatment. This amounts to 'filling out' the narrative of the patient, trying to find out more salient details – as would be expected in the care-based approaches. Having been given the opportunity to discuss these, and having been given a sympathetic explanation of the point of pressure-area care, the patient hopefully agrees to have the treatment. This is a much more desirable way to implement a principle-based approach to nursing ethics. And the expression chosen here to characterize the approach is that the principles are implemented in a manner which is infused with care. (Of course, if the patient refuses the treatment, then the approach defended here entails respect for that decision too.)

Finally, could this position of a principle-based line infused with care help in relation to the difficulties raised by consideration of suicidal patients? Regrettably, it would seem that it cannot. This is due to the fact that, in the position, although the principle-based line is implemented in a way which is infused with care, it remains the case that principles bear ultimate moral weight in decision-making. Hence, in interactions with suicidal people, the principle-based approach infused with care would entail broaching the encounter in a way analogous to the approach of nurse B in the last example. That is, the nurse ought to consider the patient's position and try to engage the patient in discussion of the feelings and so on, which prompt the suicidal intentions. It should again be stressed that this is a somewhat uncomfortable conclusion to draw.

Conclusion

We began this chapter with a brief description of and response to Clouser and Gert's challenge to principle-based ethics. We then turned to look in greater depth at care-based approaches. Considerable time was spent describing the first and most radical version such approaches, that developed by Carol Gilligan. As we saw, although there are some important points to be drawn from the approach, it seems vulnerable to criticism. More recent versions of care-based ethics do not offer anything sufficiently distinct from the principle-based approach developed here to warrant their acceptance. Towards the close of the chapter an approach which remains principle-based but which includes a key place for care was set out. The role of care in the approach is not straight-forward, because as well as the ordinary language use of the term care (as in 'Nurse A is uncaring') the term 'care' is being used in the more technical way described by Noddings and recruited above (i.e., in which to care is to try to assess what is in the best interests of the patient). The term care was also employed in the way that Gastmans describes, as a general background because of which moral problems come to our attention. We saw how care can be part of the principle-based approach to ensure that it is employed in a caring as opposed to a callous manner. Having set out the approach it would be helpful to try to show further how it might work in practice. We turn attention now to some ethical issues arising from developments in the so-called 'new genetics' to try to illustrate how the approach being proposed here might apply to them.

Chapter 6

Applying the 'Principles Infused with Care' Approach in the Context of Genetics

In this chapter, an introduction is provided, with the use of three important case examples, to some problems in nursing ethics which stem from developments in genetics. In order to illustrate the approach being developed in this book, we will apply the approach to them.

Following a review of some typical kinds of issues stemming from developments in genetics, the chapter focuses on three case examples to which we apply the approach we have been developing in the book. The examples involve (a) prenatal genetic screening, (b) confidentiality and hereditary disease, and (c) a decision to opt for pre-emptive radical surgery on the basis of genetic information provided about the risk of developing cancer. The first example, in particular, will involve a detailed analysis to try to illustrate further the way the approach can be applied to a practical ethical problem in nursing – in this case, one arising from the prenatal genetic diagnosis of a foetus with Down's syndrome.

It was decided to include a chapter on genetics due to the impact that developments in genetics have had on health care generally over the last 20 years or so. These include relatively exotic issues such as the rightness or wrongness of human reproductive cloning, and the possibilities for the genetic enhancement (Agar, 2004) of human beings, to issues such as the following:

- the selection of foetuses for implantation in the context of IVF on the basis of their genetic constitution (either because of their lack of a specific disease-causing gene, or because of their genetic match to an existing sibling – so-called 'saviour siblings' (Sheldon and Wilkinson, 2004),

- the screening and termination of foetuses because of the presence of a genetic anomaly in the foetus,

- the availability of gene therapy for certain kinds of genetic conditions (e.g., cystic fibrosis),

- the accumulation of knowledge about the genetic make-up of the population for health policy purposes,

- the possibility of screening of employees (or potential employees) for genetic predisposition to disease,

- the commercial availability of self-testing kits for diseases with a genetic causal factor,

- decisions made by people on the basis of predictive genetic screening to have drastic surgery (e.g., the removal of breasts and womb; see decision taken by two sisters of a woman diagnosed with breast cancer http://news.bbc.co.uk/1/hi/england/south_yorkshire/7189404.stm),

- problems of confidentiality arising from transmission and inheritability of genetic diseases and other uses (e.g., testing paternity),

- geneticization (viewing people solely in terms of their genetic make-up), and

- misunderstanding of information about the role of genetic factors in the causation of disease.

This is not an exhaustive list, but it gives an indication of the scope of ethical problems raised by some of the developments in genetics. To show that these are considered relevant to nursing we can point to the establishment of the International Society of Nurses in Genetics (see Cox, 2004; also www.geneticnurse.com), and numerous papers regarding the role of nurses in practice issues arising from developments in genetics. These have arisen, for example, in midwifery where midwives might be asked for advice regarding the prenatal testing of foetuses for genetic anomalies such as Down's syndrome, or spina bifida (see Metcalfe and Burton, 2003). Health visitors might also be asked for information regarding genetically caused diseases by parents of children referred for genetic investigations (Barr and McConkey, 2006). Also, a plausible case has been made for the expansion of nurse genetic counsellors (by Westwood, et al., 2006), and generally it is feasible that nurses might be asked for advice by patients about any of the issues listed above. Given that general outline of the rationale for including discussion of ethical issues in genetics, let us turn now to our first case example.

Case one: Prenatal screening for Down's syndrome

As indicated, it is not possible to discuss all the issues listed, so I will focus on just three of them, on the assumption that these will be of the kind most familiar to nursing staff. The first issue is one in the context of prenatal screening for Down's syndrome.

Janet and her husband David have decided to have a third child. Their existing children are aged 9 and 14, and as Janet is approaching her mid-thirties the couple have decided that a third child would complete their family. Janet suspects she is pregnant and contacts her local GP surgery which arranges for a midwife to come and visit her. During the meeting the midwife makes Janet aware of the option of having a blood test, later in the pregnancy, to test for the possibility of any genetic anomalies present in the foetus, in particular spina bifida and Down's syndrome. After discussion of the nature of the test, and of what the test might show, Janet agrees to have the test at the recommended stage during her pregnancy (16 weeks gestation). The day comes around and Janet has the blood test (the so-called 'triple test'). A week or so later Janet learns that, unfortunately the results of the test indicate that her baby has a higher than normal risk of having Down's syndrome (a positive result would indicate a greater than 1:250 chance of the baby having Down's syndrome). Both Janet's consultant and her midwife explain the significance of the test results to her. They explain that the tests do not show unequivocally that the baby will have Down's syndrome, merely that there is a higher than normal risk of that being so. It is explained to Janet that, if she agrees, and wanted to undergo it, it would be possible for her to have another test, amniocentesis, which would this time provide a definitive diagnosis. The information from the further test would show whether or not the baby has Down's syndrome (DS).

Janet and David discuss the situation and feel that although they would be delighted to have a healthy baby, they do not feel they could cope with a disabled child. So they opt to have the further, diagnostic test. After going this through this, the test shows that the baby does indeed have DS. Janet and David discuss this latest news and between them decide that their original feelings have not changed and that, as they do not want to have a disabled child, Janet should opt to have a termination of pregnancy. This is so even though by this stage Janet has been pregnant for approximately 22 weeks. Following further discussion with her midwife and doctor, an appointment is made for Janet to have the pregnancy terminated.

Once at the abortion clinic, Janet starts to have reservations and makes these known to the nurse who is taking her through the process of what will happen to her at the clinic. Janet asks the nurse if she is doing the right thing, and asks the nurse what she would do in the same situation.

This is clearly an important moral problem for the nurse, and of course for Janet. But let us focus on the nurse. How should she respond? If the nurse takes the moral dimension of the situation seriously, then she might consider how the principle-based approach applies to it. It is unrealistic to expect the nurse to go through the approach exhaustively in the way in which we can now, but to respond to the problem from that perspective one would open up at least the following areas for discussion.

To respect the autonomy of Janet, as we have heard, would involve respecting her decision. The fact that she is at the clinic after such a lengthy process suggests at least that her decision to have a termination of pregnancy is not one she has taken on a whim without much prior thought. So if Janet had intended to pursue the termination without any hesitation, to respect her autonomy would be to respect her chosen course of action. But as seen, now Janet appears not to be so sure about what she wants. Given this it seems appropriate to try to explore whether or not Janet actually wants to go through with the termination. So to try to do this would involve asking Janet what she thinks about the situation, whether or not she has any reservations, and if so what they are. This is all part of trying to respect the autonomy of Janet in a caring way: trying to see things from her perspective as much as possible, which involves, in turn, trying to clarify just what her view is.

It is worth pausing to consider also that the autonomy of other parties too may be relevant to Janet's decision. We have heard that her husband supports the decision to terminate the pregnancy. Let us suppose that he is still of this opinion, that he is more strongly convinced than Janet seems to be that the right thing to do is to end the pregnancy. To respect his autonomy would be to go ahead with the termination. So respecting his autonomy seems to count in favour of one course of action, but one which the main protagonist has reservations about.

In such a situation, in which there is such a conflict of two autonomous wills, it is Janet's decision which carries most moral weight from the nurse's perspective. This is because, as discussed previously, there are limits to the extent to which one is obliged to respect the autonomy of others. A striking illustration of this is when one person wants to exercise their autonomy in a way which seriously impugns the autonomy of another. To override Janet's autonomy in favour of that of her husband looks very difficult to justify. For, if it was clear that she really *did* want to proceed with the pregnancy, she would be being compelled to undergo a termination against her wishes, and that looks close to impossible to defend.

So it is clear that the autonomously expressed opinion of David contributes importantly to the moral dimension of the situation. His view is relevant even if not ultimately, the most weighty from the moral perspective. If his view does indeed conflict with that of Janet it adds a further layer of complexity to the situation as the nurse has to judge which view, from the moral perspective, is the one she should respect. In other words, although the principle of respect for autonomy obliges the nurse to respect the autonomy of others, it does not by itself show whose autonomy should be respected. Reflection on the conditions which limit respect for autonomy will help to guide the nurse in such a conflict. One set of limits, as we saw, are presented by the autonomy of others. Thus if respecting the autonomy of David impugns the autonomy of Janet, there are grounds to consider giving greater weight to the views of Janet than to those of David in this specific type of circumstance.

Why is this? Why could it not be argued that the 'weightings' should be the other way around? Thus suppose Janet becomes convinced that she does want to continue with the pregnancy. Respect for her autonomy includes respect for that view. But this then conflicts with David's autonomous view. Thus his autonomy is impinged upon, not respected. One way to try to illustrate the case for giving greatest weight to Janet's view over David's is to consider that one of the most important ways in which we respect the autonomy of others is to respect their decisions about what should happen to their own bodies. Thus we might implore a friend not to have their beautifully long hair cut short, because we enjoy the sight of their looking so beautiful. But the hairdresser would be perfectly right to respect our friend's autonomously expressed desire to have it cut than to respect our autonomously expressed desire for the hair to remain long. The 'weightings' in that trivial example also apply in the situation that Janet and David hypothetically find themselves in. Our entitlement to have our autonomy respected applies most strongly in relation to matters so intimately concerned with our own bodies that it would be very difficult to override a person's autonomously expressed desire to forgo a medical intervention because another person wanted them to have the intervention (in our example the intervention would be the termination of pregnancy).

Having made this point, there are some situations in which overriding a person's autonomous desire to do something with their body can be defended. A graphic example would be if someone stood in front of a fire exit during a fire in a building and refused to move. In such a situation their autonomous decision to stand where they like can be overridden because their exercise of autonomy in that manner seriously jeopardizes the autonomy of the other people who are trapped in the room. But of course, the Janet and David situation is not like this. David's life is not obviously endangered or harmed by Janet's decision – though he is affected by it, perhaps adversely. What significance would any such distress have that was caused to David by Janet's decision to pursue the pregnancy?

A way to illustrate this is to consider the autonomy of another group of people relevant to Janet's decision, whether this is to terminate the pregnancy or continue it. The group I am thinking of here are people with Down's syndrome themselves. In 2003 a group of people with intellectual disabilities gatecrashed a conference on prenatal screening techniques (Aspis and Souza, 2003). The intended audience for the conference were health care professionals. The intellectually disabled people had written to the organizers to ask if they could be given a space in the conference programme, but this was refused. One of the points they made during their protest was that the very existence and promotion of screening programmes for the kinds of conditions they had sent a negative message to them about the legitimacy of their existence. Thus one speaker had Down's syndrome. In a context in which prenatal screening programmes for Down's syndrome have expanded it would be reasonable for that speaker to view the conference in something like the following terms.

> The purpose of this conference is to try to make even less likely than it currently is that people like me will come into existence. You would prefer it if I had not 'got through the net', so to speak, and escaped the systems of prenatal screening which are currently in place. This says to me that my life is not valued, nor are those of people like me. Because of these things, I interpret these prenatal screening programmes as sending a hurtful message to me to the effect that everyone would be happier if I had never existed. But, nonetheless, I do exist and I have a worthwhile life. You should think about that.

The conference protesters did not use these exact words but the above passage conveys the spirit of their concerns.

Two kinds of points can be drawn from this discussion. The first helps to reinforce what has already been said regarding conflicting autonomous opinions. Just as it is not plausible to think that David's view about their pregnancy carries more moral weight than Janet's, the same is true of the protesters against prenatal screening. Their opinion would be that Janet ought not to undergo prenatal screening, but this in itself does not show that Janet's request for such screening should be denied, provided that it is an autonomous request.

The second point that the protesters' example raises is that of the place of obligations of non-maleficence. The protesters could point out that their objection to screening is not simply that in their view it should not take place. They can point to the distress that the existence of such programmes causes to them. So, it may be said, the harms caused to them by decisions such as that taken by Janet, and others in the same position, outweigh any rights Janet has to exercise her autonomy in this specific type of choice. This kind of objection to prenatal screening has in fact become known as the 'expressivist objection' because of the harm conveyed to disabled people by decisions to terminate pregnancies because of the presence of a genetic or structural anomaly in the foetus (see Buchanan, Brock et al., 2000; Edwards, 2005). Obviously, there is rarely, if ever, any intention to cause harm to groups of people with disabilities by women who opt to take up pre-natal screening procedures of the kind undergone by Janet. But regard-less of intent, the point made by the protesters in the example above seems well made and one can understand why they might be opposed to such practices.

However, what significance does that harm have? We know that there are limits to the extent to which obligations to respect auton-omy apply, does this case present such a limit? In other words, is this a situation in which a person (Janet) is exercising her autonomy in a way which goes beyond the limits to which her autonomy should be respected?

To see that it does not, consider the following analogy. Suppose you are not a vegetarian but you have friends who are. You invite them to your house for a meal and cook them a vegetarian dish. For yourself, however, you cook a meat dish. When the time comes to eat, your friends express disgust at the fact that you are eating meat. They are clearly offended by your choice. You might decide to carry on eating the meat, or you might save it until after they've gone. But what seems plain is that the choice is yours to make. The harm caused to your friends by your choice of menu is morally relevant, but it is not weight-ier than your own autonomously arrived at choice to eat meat. So in this 'meat eater' case, it looks like an entitlement to make and enact an autonomous desire to eat meat is weightier than the harm caused to the vegetarian friends. If this is accepted, it suggests that obligations to respect autonomy are morally weightier than obligations not to harm others in at least some cases.

To expand on this point, we saw that the autonomy of others presents a limit on the extent to which we are entitled to exercise our own autonomy, and also the extent to which we are obliged to respect the autonomy of others. The most graphic illustrations of cases in which such limits are breached include murder and assault. Such acts constitute serious breaches of the autonomy others and in large part this is what accounts for their wrongness. The two examples we have been looking at so far – 'the protesters' and the 'vegetarian friends' cases – do not involve such serious transgressions of autonomy. Yet the harm caused to the protesters and to the friends is plainly mor-ally relevant. So why does not this count for so much, that the harm done to them is of greater moral significance than the entitlement to make autonomous choices and to act on them? Let us use the 'friends' example to illustrate why, since this is perhaps the less serious of the issues raised in the two examples. An explanation is that by choosing to eat meat, one does not prevent one's friends from pursuing their own vegetarian choice. So although one might upset them by one's choices and thus harm them, one is not transgressing their autonomy in any way which prevents them from pursuing their own 'life plan', as this idea was explained in Chapter 3 above. They could simply leave your house, and choose to socialize only with fellow vegetarians. So your choice to eat meat would not intrude upon their autonomy in the way in which assaulting one of them would. This looks even more obvious in the nursing context. So suppose one asks a patient what they would like to eat, and they opt for the meat dish. A patient in the next bed, who happens to be vegetarian, expresses disgust at the fact that anyone could eat meat. If the first patient really wants the meat dish, the nurse is under a stronger obligation to respect his autonomous desire than to withhold the meat dish from him because of the offence this causes to his neighbour.

I think the same kind of analysis applies even in the 'protesters' example, with one specific qualification. Suppose Janet's decisions to undergo screening really are autonomous ones. Thus she is not being pressured into doing something she is unsure about either by her husband David or by the health care professionals she has come into contact with so far. Her decisions do not in themselves impugn the autonomy of the protesters or other intellectually disabled people. They can pursue their own 'life plan' and make their own choices irrespective of Janet's decision. And imagine it was claimed that the harm caused to the protesters by Janet's decision is of greater moral significance than Janet's views regarding what should happen to her body. It would be extremely difficult to mount a persuasive case to the effect that the harms endured by the protesters are of such a magnitude that they warrant preventing Janet from undergoing the screening procedures she has autonomously chosen to undergo.

The qualification mentioned above, though, concerns this very point: is Janet's decision to undergo screening procedures an autonomous one? Even if we set aside the possibilities of her having been pressurized by other parties into having the tests, the protesters discussed above might argue that Janet's decision is not autonomous (see e.g., Ockleford, Berryman and Hsu, 2003). They might say this because it may be that Janet has a mistaken conception of the nature of the screened for conditions. Thus suppose Janet does eventually decide to proceed and to terminate the pregnancy because the foetus has Down's syndrome. But suppose her understanding of what kind of life is possible for a person with Down's syndrome is deeply mistaken. She would not be unusual if that were the case. A journalist recounted her experiences of making the same kind of decision which Janet is involved with in our example. She was informed, though, that a life with Down's syndrome will inevitably involve high levels of suffering due to medical problems associated with the condition. She was also told that any child she had with Down's syndrome would be wholly dependent upon her for all its life (Loach, 2003). This is misleading information. So if Janet does indeed have a mistaken conception of life with Down's syndrome, then it is important for those involved in her care to try to ensure that her conception of that condition is an informed one, otherwise the decision is not autonomous (recall our discussion of this in Chapter 3 above). In our case example this may be one aspect of the situation which the nurse might try to explore.

So far then we have focused on autonomy and harms, and we have spoken of Janet herself, her husband and others that might be affected by Janet's decisions. But we have not mentioned the perspective of her existing children. Their children Ben aged 14 and Bridget aged 9 are also affected by the situation and their opinions and the effects on them are plainly relevant to the moral dimensions of it.

To do justice to their autonomy, it will be important at least to ask them how they would feel about a new family member, one who has Down's syndrome. It is interesting to pose the question about limits to autonomy in relation to Janet's existing children. We saw above in discussion of the autonomy of David, the protesters and the vegetarian friends that it looked difficult to justify placing limits on Janet's autonomy as far as decisions regarding her own body are concerned, even though the decisions she takes might affect others adversely. A way to try to specify such limits is via the notion of a 'life plan', or set of autonomous choices. Thus since Janet's decision to eat meat need not disrupt the life plan or her vegetarian friends, there is no obligation on her part to change her behaviour (at least on those grounds). Similarly, the same is true in relation to Janet's decision to have prenatal screening and the effect this has on the protesters. But what about her own children? Plausibly, any decision Janet makes to proceed with the pregnancy will have an impact upon Ben and Bridget. Some research suggests that families in which there is a disabled child are more susceptible to family breakdown and other problems, including poverty (see Reinders, 2000). The decision taken by the journalist mentioned above to terminate her pregnancy stemmed in part from fears about the negative impact on her existing child were she to have a disabled baby (as she saw the situation). Suppose, then, that Ben and Bridget thought Janet should not have the baby and that Janet thought she should. Would Janet's entitlement to make her own decisions about her own life have such a severe impact upon that of Ben and Bridget that their 'life plans' or their choices would seriously be adversely affected?

Again it seems to me that the answer to this question is 'no', and that Janet would be entitled to expect her autonomous decision to prevail over that of her children. The reasons are these. Suppose it becomes evident that having this third child is an important part of her life plan and is not something that she has rushed into without thought. Also, it seems reasonable to assume that, as the parent of Ben and Bridget she is sufficiently clear that she can make sure they are cared for and not neglected in such a way that their prospects or their lives within the family are impugned by their new sibling. In addition, it is not reasonable to assume that their new sibling would inevitably impair the quality of family experiences for the two existing children. Although there is research suggesting increases in divorce rates and family break-up in families with a disabled child, there are other reports which present a more positive story (see Reinders, 2000). Also, of course, one can point out too that a third child, with or without a disability, will inevitably have some impact upon the existing family members. So, overall, if Janet's decision is indeed autonomously taken, there do seem these reasons to judge that it should prevail in the face of opposition from her two existing children. If things were different, however, and if it could be shown to be very likely that adding a new child to the existing family would have a seriously damaging effect on the family, it looks as though that would be a decision which is difficult to justify. Such a decision could fall within the range of decisions which are those in which one person exercises their autonomy in a way which seriously impugns the autonomy of another. And 'seriously impugns' means that it significantly reduces the likelihood that her children's capacity to pursue what I have labelled a 'life plan' of even minimal quality.

So far then we have mentioned the autonomy of many of the parties involved in Janet's decision: her husband, the protesters, and to Janet's existing children. Turn now to consider obligations of non-maleficence.

Let us think about Janet first. It is possible that undergoing a termination may cause her considerable harm. Not simply the harm endured during the process itself, but it is reported that many women experience varying levels of psychological distress when they look back upon their decisions to terminate a pregnancy (see e.g., Korenromp et al., 2007). So there are risks of harm to Janet if she opts to terminate the pregnancy.

Similarly, there are risks of harm to her if she pursues the pregnancy. She will experience some distress during the birth itself of course, and some discomfort prior to that too. Moreover, if her decision runs against that of her husband this may cause some friction between them, and thus lead to a further set of harms. So there are risks of significant harms whichever option Janet decides upon.

With reference to her husband David, if it remains the case that he would prefer the pregnancy to be terminated, then any distress caused by a decision to continue the pregnancy would be morally relevant. He might also suggest that there are other harms he is likely to have to endure, such as reduced economic freedom due to the additional family member, less time for leisure and less time for spending with Ben and Bridget.

We have already discussed the harms that might befall Ben and Bridget and those that might be experienced by the protesters above, or anyone with similar sympathies. These can be considered in the context of Janet's opting to terminate or pursue the pregnancy. The protesters will not be harmed by Janet's decision if she opts to continue the pregnancy, but could be if she decides to terminate it.

The same kind of analysis that was undertaken in relation to conflicts of autonomy between the protesters and Janet can be applied here. Any harms caused to the protesters by Janet's decision are not outweighed by her entitlement to make such an important decision herself. With reference to Ben and Bridget, although this is more difficult to assess, I think the same analysis applies there too. This is because it is not known that they will experience any harms due to a decision to proceed with the pregnancy.

So far the relevance of any harms endured by the foetus has not been mentioned. Let us assume that the foetus will not be harmed by coming into existence. The disabilities associated with DS are not on the same scale as other, much more serious genetic diseases such as Lesch Nyhan disease or Tay Sach's disease. These latter two conditions typically involve much suffering and death at a young age. This is not the case with DS. So there does seem a sense in which the foetus is harmed if terminated. (I am assuming that the foetus is not harmed in the actual process of termination – that this is done in such a way as to cause no experienced distress to the foetus.) Arguably, the harm done lies in the deprivation of a future (see Marquis, 1989). Obviously this line of argument is only relevant to our example if Janet is considering opting for a termination. So let's suppose she is. Can we weigh the harm done to the foetus against Janet's own autonomous decision to terminate the pregnancy?

When we tried to weigh obligations to respect Janet's autonomous decisions regarding the pregnancy against harms to third parties we appealed to the idea of a life plan, something a person autonomously chooses. If a decision by one person severely jeopardizes the capacity of another to pursue their life plan, then this may present a limit to the extent to which one is obliged to respect the autonomy of the person. Hence, if A embarks upon a course of action which severely jeopardizes B's capacity to pursue a life plan, then A's action may not be justifiable. It has to be asked, then, whether a decision by Janet to terminate the pregnancy is an example of such a decision.

One way to respond to this is to state that a decision to terminate would indeed be such a decision and so would illustrate another limit to the extent to which we are obliged to respect the autonomy of others. For, in choosing to terminate the foetus, one removes the possibility of its ever being in a position to formulate a life plan. However, there are at least two strong rejoinders to this proposal. The first is that in our Janet and David scenario the discussion so far has only concerned existing autonomous people and so the discussion involving the foetus is importantly different from what we have discussed so far. This is because there is no autonomy present in the foetus to 'thwart' so to speak. To illustrate this, suppose that Janet agrees to fund a school trip for Bridget, one that she is desperate to go on. Then, Janet changes her mind and decides she will use the money to buy a new dress for herself. Bridget's plan to go on the school trip is thus disrupted by Janet's change of mind. But there is no similar way in which a foetus could have a plan thwarted since, of course, it is incapable of forming plans.

The second response is to remind ourselves of the importance of respecting Janet's own autonomy. If she were to be prevented from having a termination which she had autonomously chosen, that would be grave violation of respect for her autonomy. She would, effectively, be being compelled to go through a lengthy, uncomfortable, possibly painful ordeal.

These two points illustrate the implausibility of a claim that Janet's autonomy is constrained by that of the foetus to such an extent that considerations relating to its autonomy outweigh Janet's own choices.

Having analysed the situation in relation to principles of autonomy, beneficence and non-maleficence, it is necessary to consider the principle of justice. If we focus on the issue of health care resources, it might be argued that the best use of such resources would be to terminate the foetus. One may be drawn to such a conclusion if one thinks that a baby with Down's syndrome is likely to generate considerable costs to the NHS. One might think this because of the medical problems which are often associated with DS, such as circulatory problems and early-onset dementia. However, this financial case might not be compelling. Alderson (2001), for example, has queried the cost-effectiveness of prenatal screening programmes for DS since no research has compared the costs of the programme against the costs of supporting people who live with DS. Suppose, though, it could be shown that the costs to the public purse in terms of additional social, educational and health services are greater when a child is born with DS compared with the overall costs incurred when a healthy baby is born. It would be difficult to make such a calculation because it is hard to predict what the economic contribution to a country generated by a person will be. But, again, for the sake of argument let it be accepted that, overall, it costs more to support a decent life for someone with DS than it does to support a healthy child. Do these 'justice-based' considerations constitute a limit to the extent to which there is an obligation to respect a person's choice to give birth to child with DS (or indeed to knowingly give birth to any child likely to have a greater than average amount of health problems combined with a lower than average contribution to the economy in the form of tax contributions)?

Some commentators argue that if one knowingly brings into the world a baby with significant health and social needs, then this is only defensible if one puts in place funding to cover these anticipated additional costs (see Buchanan, Brock et al., 2000). Thus on such a view, justice obliges one not to impinge upon others to pay for foreseeable expenditures which one is unable to cover oneself. A view such as this is very similar to the conception of justice proposed by Nozick and described above (Chapter 3). According to that we have no obligation to pay taxes to maintain the well-being of others who are unable to support themselves. So if we adopted this kind of Nozickian conception of justice, Janet's situation would be such that if she decided to pursue the pregnancy, she could not rely upon any additional financial support she or her child might need. Given the correlation between DS and other medical problems one can imagine that such justice-based considerations might steer Janet towards the option of termination of the pregnancy since David and she are not especially wealthy. However, of course, Janet is not making her decision in a Nozickian context.

Recall also, that we rejected a Nozickian conception of justice in favour of something less extreme, a broadly Rawlsian account. Within this, there is scope to take taxable income from some people and redistribute it to others. Such monies can be used for health, education and social support, amongst other things. The point of such schemes of taxation is to try to ensure that all citizens of the state can lead a life of at least minimal decency. This means trying to ensure, at least, that the basic needs of citizens are met. Thus, needs for shelter, food, health care and education are undertaken to be met by the state in this Rawlsian conception of justice. In a context such as that, one close to the current situation in the United Kingdom, for the short term at least Janet could expect that if her child were to be in need of additional support, at least for basic needs, then it would be available to her.

As mentioned at the start of this analysis of Janet's situation through the lens of the principles, it is not feasible to expect the nurse with whom she is talking to to conduct the kind of analysis that we have done so far in this chapter. But the analysis presented gives an illustration of what a full treatment might look like. In the actual situation, the nurse's pressing concern is to try to ensure that Janet's decision is autonomous, which is to say that it is based on accurate information, and is not coerced. Respecting Janet's autonomy requires respecting her decision, unless this radically conflicts with Janet's best interests as the nurse sees them. If this is the case, then the nurse should think about the same kind of strategy we described in relation to the patient in need of pressure-area care, thus the nurse should implement a 'principles infused with care' approach.

Case two: A request to keep genetic information confidential

The next situation to be discussed is as follows:

Helen is 20 years old. She has become increasingly concerned about her mother's health. Over the past 10 months or so, her mother Alice, has become increasingly forgetful, and has had several minor accidents in the house, dropping dishes and various ornaments; she has also become very irritable which is in contrast to her usual, calm self. Because of these changes in her mother, Helen has persuaded Alice to make an appointment at her local GP's surgery. Alice does this and having spoken to the receptionist has made an appointment to see Heather, the practice nurse. Alice confides to Heather that her own mother had Huntington's disease, but she herself was never informed that she had it. She explained that due to her fears that she might have the disease, she could never bring herself to have a test to find this out. However, Alice is aware that her health problems might be the manifestations of Huntington's disease. She is also aware that this means she is likely to have passed the disease on to her daughter Helen. Worse still, she believes that Helen might be pregnant and, if so, that Helen could have unwittingly passed on the Huntington's gene to her own baby. Alice begs the nurse to keep all this to herself. If she (the nurse) must record the details of their conversation, that is fine but it is imperative that her daughter is not told. ' what good would it do?' Alice asks the nurse. That question seems a good one since there is no cure for Huntington's disease and keeping the information from Helen would spare her the anguish that learning about the disease is sure to cause her.

Here, then, is a terrible situation. One person, Alice, has entered into the early stages of a fatal, severely debilitating hereditary disease and is likely to die within 5 to 10 years, perhaps sooner. Before that she will lose any capacity to live independently. Her daughter will certainly have the same disease. She may not begin to experience any symptoms of it for twenty years or so. Moreover, it turns out that she is pregnant and if she has the gene which causes Huntington's disease so will her child.

Let us begin with Alice's request that the information about her illness be withheld from Helen. How strong is the obligation to respect Alice's request here? We need to ask whether respecting Alice's autonomy would lead to a significant breach of (in this case) Helen's autonomy.

An argument that it would indeed count as such a situation looks fairly easy to construct. As outlined in Chapter 3 above, it is reasonable to think that the principle of respect for autonomy includes obligations to give people relevant information about their lives. This is necessary for them to be 'self-governing'. If we deprive information from people we reduce the extent to which they can lead their lives in the way they want to, pursue their 'life plan' as it was put earlier. In this current case, for example, if she wanted to, Helen could terminate her pregnancy. As things stand currently she would not entertain this option as she is looking forward to the birth of her child. Even when given the awful news about Huntington's disease she might still decide to proceed with the pregnancy. But at least then that would have been her choice, made in full knowledge of the facts. These are the kinds of autonomy-related considerations prompted by Alice's request. It looks, at first sight anyway, as though respect for Alice's autonomy would impugn too much the autonomy of Helen for a pressing case to be made in favour of respecting it.

However, we noted in our discussion of paternalism (Chapter 4 above) that on occasion, paternalistic acts can be defensible. Might this be just such an occasion? As Alice pointed out to the nurse, Huntington's disease is incurable. If Helen is given the facts she will be devastated. Her mother is dying, and she too has the same disease which will inevitably cause her to die in the same way. Not only that, she is pregnant and has a terrible decision to make of her own: whether or not to terminate her current pregnancy. And of course, perhaps overshadowing all this is the knowledge that her mother has kept all this information from her. This is obviously likely to raise questions in Helen's mind about how her mother has handled the situation, and may even cause her to wonder if there are any other things about her family that have been kept from her too. Thus, because it is obvious that passing on the information to Helen will cause her great harm, Heather might wonder whether she should indeed respect Alice's request. Moreover, Heather might recall that her own NMC Code draws attention to the importance of confidentiality.

Although this might look a persuasive case in favour of respecting Alice's wish, recall our discussion of paternalism (Chapter 4). It looks as though it will be highly problematic, at best, to justify the kind of paternalism that withholding the information from Helen would require. Recall too that for Heather's decision to be paternalistic, the primary rationale for withholding the information from her must be to protect her from harm (in this case). So Heather must be convinced that protecting Helen from the news about the diagnosis is the right thing to do because that it is the option which will cause her least harm: in Benjamin and Curtis's terms, Heather is acting on Helen's behalf by withholding the information from her, but is not acting at Helen's behest – because Helen is thus far ignorant of the real cause of her mother's illness, and its implications for her own life.

On Benjamin and Curtis's analysis, though, if Helen is capable of understanding the information – if she meets the 'autonomy condition' – then paternalism will not be justified. This is so even if it is agreed that withholding the information from Helen is the least harmful option. And that too is far from clear. This is because if the information is withheld from Helen, she will give birth to her baby without knowing the health consequences of this for her child. And, as her own mother's illness progresses it seems likely that she will be made aware of the true nature of the illness and its implications for her. So even the claim that withholding the information from Helen is the least harmful option can be challenged.

There is no need for us to analyse this present situation in the same depth that we analysed the previous case. This is because here the main issues can be set out in terms of autonomy and paternalism, and as seen, it looks as though Heather's obligations to Helen outweigh the importance of respecting the autonomy of Alice. To fail to inform Heather would be a serious failure to respect her autonomy.

To add something about the application of the principles being infused with care in this case, recall that to do this involves trying to put oneself in the position of the other person, as far as one can, and trying to make some assessment of what is in their best interests. So suppose Heather tries to see the situation, as far as she is able to. First she will appreciate why Alice wants the information withheld from Helen. As Alice says, Helen herself will be greatly distressed by this and yet there will be no chance of a cure. So what good can come of informing Helen? Also, even if Helen is pregnant, Alice might think she should still proceed with the pregnancy rather than terminate it. It is still possible to have forty years of good quality life (sometimes more) with Huntington's disease, and the same will be true of Helen's child. Who knows? with luck a cure or some effective treatment may have been developed by the time Helen or her child begin to develop the symptoms of the disease. So doing one's best to assume Alice has really thought about her decision, Heather might be led to these kinds of points. She now has to try to think about whether, given these points, it is in Alice's best interests that the information is kept from Helen. That it might not be can be indicated by the points we mentioned above: in particular the point that Helen might be devastated that Alice kept this information from her, and may feel that it is up to her to decide whether to continue with the pregnancy. Also, as mentioned, Helen will find out almost inevitably what is wrong with Alice as her disease progresses. By then she may have already had her child and so an important choice has been denied her by her mother (and by Heather and the health care team of course). Given these considerations Heather might then try to explore more fully with Alice the reasons why she thinks it best to keep the information from Helen, and draw attention to the points we have just made. Of course, Alice might still think it best that the information is kept from Helen. But if so, as explained above, this looks like one confidence it will not be possible to keep.

Case three: A decision to have radical surgery on the basis of genetic information

The last case to be described in this chapter is one that was recently reported in the news (BBC, 15/1/08).

It has been included for discussion since it raises issues that are likely to become increasingly prevalent. The case involves three sisters who all underwent radical surgery, two of them for preventative purposes only.

In January 2008 it emerged that three sisters had all chosen to undergo radical surgery, specifically, each sister had their breasts and womb removed. This was because one of the sisters, Michelle, had been diagnosed with breast cancer. Moreover, she discovered there was a family history of ovarian and breast cancer, which suggested the presence of a genetic basis of the disease. As treatment for her own cancer, Michelle had a double mastectomy and hysterectomy. Because of the medical history of their family, and also because of Michelle's positive diagnosis, her two sisters decided to be tested to determine whether or not they too had the gene thought causally responsible for the cancer (BRCA1, or BRCA2). Unfortunately, the tests proved positive. After much thought, all three opted to have the radical surgery. This was the case even though two of the sisters – Joanne Kavanagh and Louise Lambert – were cancer-free at the time. So their decision was entirely precautionary. From what the sisters have said (see BBC, 15/1/08) they were fearful that the cancer might develop without them being aware of it. Hence, they were fearful that they might die as a consequence of developing the cancer. Since, as they put it, they wanted to live to see their respective children grow up they opted for the radical surgery.

It is easy to imagine that during the course of their consultations with various health care professionals, one of the sisters might have confessed to having some doubts about whether or not she was doing the right thing. She might raise this with a nurse in the relevant oncology unit. In one way, this looks a straightforward problem. If the sister wants the radical treatment, then to respect her autonomy is to respect that wish. But recall our discussion of autonomous choice in Chapter 3 above. Are the conditions necessary for this met?

One difficulty with this kind of choice is that some understanding of probability of risk is necessary. So it would be important for the nurse to try to ensure that the sister is aware that the presence of the gene does not mean the sister will inevitably develop either breast or ovarian cancer. Obviously, if the sister's decision to opt for surgery is based on such misunderstanding, it fails to meet the conditions for autonomous decision-making.

In the same vein, if the sister is unaware of the other possible options, then this too would show the decision not to be autonomous. For example, another option would have been to have her condition closely monitored to check for cancerous growths. From what the sisters say it looks as though they were certainly aware of this other option. But less is known about their understanding of the relationship between the presence of the gene and the manifestation of the cancer.

A further possible option that the nurse might want to exclude is the possibility of coercion. Suppose one of the two sisters yet to develop the disease is very determined that the best course of action is for them both to have the radical surgery. It would be important to be sure that the sister is making the decision herself and does not feel coerced into making it – into going along with what her sister thinks is best, simply because she does not want to upset her sister during what is, obviously, a stressful period. In other words, it is important to try to ensure the decision is free from *controlling* influences, which (recall) is not to require that it is free from any influences whatsoever.

With reference to the nurse's obligations of beneficence and non-maleficence, this looks like a situation in which there is such a personal element in the weighing of these that it would be difficult for the nurse to calculate which option would be in the best interests of the sister. For the sister the thought of the cancer developing whilst she is 'between' check ups, so to speak, might be so terrifying that she may be unable to lead a normal life after the test which showed the presence of the gene. So given that the option of regular check ups would prove too stressful for her, one can understand how the option of radical surgery might seem the less harmful of the two options. Additionally, of course, the removal of the breasts and womb ensures the cancer cannot develop since the bodily tissues in which it develops are removed. Given this 'personal' element in the weighing of harms and benefits, provided the decision is autonomous, the nurse's obligation would be to respect it.

As a way of trying to structure one's thinking about risk assessment, Beauchamp and Childress point out (2009, p. 224) that we can distinguish high and low levels of risk, on one hand, and major and minor levels of harm on the other. Thus an option which has a low risk of minor harm is preferable to one which involves a high risk of major harm. Consider again, then the predicament of the two sisters who were cancer-free at the time of the surgery. In their case the surgery plainly presents a high risk – a certainty in fact – of major harm. But their view, evidently, was that living with the increased risk of cancer was the greater harm to them.

Suppose, then, that the sister after having spoken with the nurse is confident that the right decision for her is indeed to proceed with the surgery. The nurse is also confident after discussion with the sister that her decision is indeed autonomous and has not been coerced: the sister is aware that the presence of the gene points only to an increased risk, not a certainty that she will develop breast or ovarian cancer, and she has not been pressured into the decision by her other sisters, or anyone else. To try to ensure the nurse's response to the situation is infused with care, she should try to assess whether the sister's decision is in conflict with the best interests of the sister. As noted above, the nurse can only attempt this. She can't view the situation exactly as the sister herself does. If the relevant considerations are those we have already set out, and if the decision of the sister is an informed one, then the decision to undergo the surgery, although extreme, is plausibly seen as being in the best interests of the sister, given her specific priorities and values.

Conclusion

So in this chapter we have highlighted a range of problems which are prompted by developments in genetics, and we have considered three specific case examples of such problems. By doing this it has been possible to illustrate more concretely how the version of principle-based approaches to ethics described here might apply to 'real-life' moral problems in nursing. Our next, and final chapter continues to do this. But it focuses on situations in which nurses themselves are facing stressful and apparently impossible ethical problems.

Chapter 7

Supererogatory Actions in the Context of Nursing

In this final chapter, the discussion is focused again on the moral principles we have discussed. Although the topic may seem somewhat abstract, it provides a further example of the way in which the principle-based approach can be used to structure thought within nursing ethics, and to aid clear thought. The chapter begins by employing the principles to help to distinguish ordinary from extraordinary moral standards. This will then help to identify a class of actions which are described as supererogatory (roughly, as will be seen, these are actions which are for the benefit of others, but which expose the actor to significant risk of harm). The question of the extent to which nurses are called upon, or even obliged to undertake such actions, will then be considered.

Before embarking on to the main body of the chapter it is important to comment upon a change that has occurred between 1994 when the first edition was being prepared, and the current situation in 2008. As readers of the first edition may recall, the situation at that time placed nurses in an impossibly difficult situation. This is because the Code in place at the time (UKCC, 1992) made it clear that nurses had a professional obligation to take action if the environment of care was such that standards of care were jeopardized. For example if circumstances were such that 'safe and appropriate care' (UKCC, 1992, clause 12) could not be provided – say, due to staff shortages or shortages of equipment – then nurses were required to act to do something to change this. The same applied, at the time, if circumstances were such that 'the health or safety of colleagues is at risk' (ibid., clause 13).

So, suppose a nurse has exhausted all available internal avenues to draw attention to such problems. The nurse might then conclude that it would be justifiable to become a 'whistleblower' and make her concerns public. This in fact, is what a well-known nurse, Graham Pink, did in 1990 (see http://society.guardian.co.uk/societyguardian/story/0,7843,1304327,00.html). As readers will be aware, Pink's actions were not well received by his hospital managers and he was suspended from duty and eventually sacked for breaching confidentiality. Moreover, at the time, The Department of Health's Management Committee stated that breaches of confidentiality '[Will] always warrant disciplinary action' (DoH, 1993, clause 8).

Thus, on the one hand, it seemed, nurses could be vulnerable to disciplinary action if they failed to maintain standards of care that were safe and therapeutic for patients. And yet, on the other hand, in some circumstances, if they took steps to try to address these concerns they could be disciplined for breaching confidentiality and lose their jobs, or at best have their career prospects severely dented.

Since those days, people have come to see the value of having a forum in which employees can draw attention to concerns about, for example, patient safety and do so anonymously. And, in the United Kingdom, the Public Interest Disclosure Act came into force in 1998. Under the terms of this, employees can raise concerns regarding dangerous practices or circumstances which constitute a danger to health and safety. A person can do this without their identity being passed on to their employer. The legislation covers all NHS employees (see Public Concern at Work). So this marks a radical difference between the period before and after the legislation. As mentioned, at the time of writing the first edition it seemed that nurses were in an impossible situation. Things seem to have changed for the better in that respect at least, which is not to say that it is easy to draw attention to poor standards of care (for more on this topic see e.g., Dooley and McCarthy, 2005, chapter 16; Wilmot, 2000).

The relevance of this to our present topic is that actions which are for the benefit of others, but which expose the actor to high risk of serious harm are sometimes described as 'supererogatory acts'. So if a nurse loses her job because of voicing concerns about levels of patient care, then such acts may well fall into that category. But let us look in more detail at the nature of supererogatory acts.

What are supererogatory acts?

Beauchamp and Childress (2009, p. 47) suggest that a distinction may be drawn between ordinary and extraordinary moral standards. They indicate that 'everyone' is bound by ordinary moral standards; but, they add, it is not the case that everyone is bound by extraordinary moral standards. But how could a distinction between ordinary and extraordinary moral standards be set out?

One way to do this is to recruit the four principles we have been discussing. For example, it can be claimed that the principles of respect for autonomy, non-maleficence and justice structure the obligations of *ordinary* moral standards; and in the context of *extraordinary* moral standards these are buttressed by additional obligations of beneficence. So for most of us we try to respect others, not harm them, and be fair, but we are not generally thought to be subject to a strong obligation to help others especially when in doing so we expose ourselves to high risk of harms. It is worth stressing that the principles which characterize ordinary moral standards refer to fairly minimal obligations. These are, of course, obligations to respect autonomy, not to harm others and to deal with others fairly.

The more demanding obligations captured by the principle of beneficence do not appear to feature among ordinary moral standards. It is considered morally acceptable to eat meat, to fail to respond to the plight of homeless people, and to fail to respond to the plight of persons in poor countries. Obviously one might think one should do these things, but there are no obvious penalties or serious moral criticisms if one does not do them.

In the context of ordinary moral standards, a distinction seems to be drawn between harming someone by omitting to help them, and harming someone by actively hurting them. Hence, although by ordinary moral standards, it is acceptable to walk past a person in need of financial aid (a person who is homeless and hungry let us say), it is not considered acceptable to strike such a person. It might, though, be contended that even in ordinary morality there is, in fact, an obligation to help the person in dire financial need – say, a homeless and hungry person. This amounts to the claim that it is widely considered a moral wrong not to help such a person. On such a view, it is held that obligations of beneficence do indeed feature in ordinary moral standards. This proposal sounds much too strong to me if it is taken to reflect a current moral consensus to the effect that it is obligatory to provide such help. But suppose that it is accepted.

Even if it is allowed that the obligations referred to by the principle of beneficence do feature among ordinary moral standards, the extent of its application is extremely limited. To see this, recall that there is a very strong obligation not to harm others by one's intentional actions, for example by striking someone. This is buttressed by the law: to strike someone who asks one for money is to break the law, but to ignore that person's request for help is not to break the law. If it is accepted that the law reflects a broad moral consensus, this illustrates the force of the kind of obligations referred to by the principle of nonmaleficence. It may be claimed that although one would not break the law if one refused to help someone who is hungry and homeless one really should try to do something to help them. Even if this consists simply in giving the person a small sum of money to spend as they choose.

Suppose this view is accepted. However, it is clear that there are limits to the obligations referred to by the principle of beneficence, even if is accepted that they do feature in ordinary moral standards. To see this we need only remind ourselves that, by ordinary moral standards, the principle of beneficence does not extend to include as obligatory acts which will benefit others if acting in such a way results in harm (or deprivation) to the actor. Hence, although it may be argued that by ordinary moral standards one is under an obligation of beneficence to the person who is homeless and hungry, it is unlikely to be maintained that one is obliged to give to the person to the extent that this will result in some suffering to oneself or to one's dependents. So, even if in ordinary morality it is the case that obligations of beneficence are recognized, these appear to be extremely limited.

Actions which are done in accordance with extraordinary moral standards are termed 'supererogatory' by Beauchamp and Childress; such acts

> are optional; [they are] neither required nor forbidden by common-morality standards. [They] exceed what the common morality demands. [They]

are intentionally undertaken to promote the welfare of others. [And they] are morally praiseworthy and good in themselves'. (2009, p. 48)

This passage, then, illustrates the defining aspects of supererogatory acts. They go beyond what is required according to ordinary moral standards and their aim is to promote the good of others. Hence, a person who acts in ways which are for the benefit of others but which expose the actor to significant risk of harm, would be said to undertake supererogatory acts. By ordinary moral standards, such sacrifices are not morally obligatory.

It should be added that within the class of supererogatory acts a further, rough, distinction can be made between actions which exemplify 'lower-level supererogation', and what is termed 'higher-level super-erogation' (Beauchamp and Childress, 2009, p. 49). An action which exhibited lower-level supererogation would be for the benefit of others but would expose the actor to low risk of harm, or incur low levels of harm. An act of high-level supererogation, obviously, would also be for the benefit of others, but would run a high risk of harm, or incur a high level of harm, to the actor.

So, it seems possible to make out the distinction between ordinary and extraordinary moral standards by invoking the four principles. Further, as we have seen, making the distinction in this way makes possible the characterization of supererogatory acts. To consider properly the context of supererogatory acts within nursing, it is necessary next to identify the parties to whom nurses do, in fact, have obligations to.

To whom do nurses have obligations?

A distinction can be made between professional duties and obligations, and moral obligations and duties. By entering into the nursing profession, nurses take on certain professional obligations and duties. These are stated in the NMC Code (2008; see Appendix): nurses have obligations to respect confidentiality, to obtain consent, to respect the religious beliefs of patients, and so on.

In addition to these professional obligations, nurses are under certain moral obligations. The point can be made that nursing is not the kind of occupation which people enter into simply for the financial rewards; rather, nursing is entered into by persons who, by and large, want to help others – want to do good. In Chapter 1, we considered

Seedhouse's (1988, p. xvii) claim that work for health is a moral endeavour. This is because health work involves striving towards an end which is deemed to constitute a 'good'; namely, the aim is to improve the health, relieve the suffering, and foster the autonomy of those who are patients and clients.

So, nurses are certainly under professional obligations (as set out in the NMC Code) and, if work for health is a moral endeavour (as it can plausibly be regarded), then nurses would seem to be under certain moral obligations. But to whom do nurses have these obligations? At least seven groups and individuals can be identified.

1. *Other nurses.* The NMC Code indicate that nurses have professional obligations to their fellow nurses. Thus it states one must treat colleagues 'fairly and without discrimination' (NMC, 2008); reference is also made to the importance of keeping colleagues who care for the same patients as oneself informed. Another clause refers to the obligation to act quickly if one thinks a patient could be harmed by one's own actions or by those of a colleague.

It is easy to illustrate the ways in which these professional obligations have their moral foundation in the various moral principles. The reference to treating colleagues fairly plainly rests upon the principle of justice; the reference to keeping colleagues informed invokes at least the principle of respect for autonomy: it is only if colleagues are in possession of relevant information that they can make informed, autonomous decisions about the care of their patients. And the reference to harm prevention rests upon the principle of non-maleficence.

2. *Patients and their relatives.* Professional obligations to promote the well-being of patients and their relatives are referred to in the NMC Code (2008). There it is stated that as a nurse one must 'Work with others to protect and promote the health and wellbeing of those in your care, their families and carers' (NMC, 2008).

The moral foundations of these professional obligations lie in the moral principles of beneficence and non-maleficence as the clauses concern promotion of benefit and the prevention of harms.

3. *Other health care professionals.* The Code states professional obligations to assist other members of the health care team. It refers to obligations to share information with colleagues, to work as part of a team, to delegate effectively and to ensure that professional standards are upheld.

It is plausible to think of these clauses as having their moral foundations in the four principles. For example, sharing information helps to ensure that patients are given the appropriate treatments, and thus are not harmed but benefited as a result of the interventions of the health care team. Sharing information can also help to guard against wasting resources: if one nurse is aware that an intervention has been carried out with a patient, there is no need for her to check that it has been done. Thus her time can be used for other opportunities to care. Keeping colleagues informed about the patients in their care helps to respect their own autonomy too. Plainly if, as a nurse, one is deprived of key information about a patient, for example concerning their diet or religion, this may adversely affect the quality of the care one can give that patient. So it is evident that these obligations to work as a team and uphold standards can all be feasibly claimed to have as their moral foundation one or other of the four principles.

4. *The general public.* The Code also states that nurses have a duty 'to uphold the reputation of your profession' (NMC, 2008). A fair interpretation of this is that, even when not officially on nursing duty, certain kinds of behaviours should not be done. Most obviously, it can be supposed, the nurse should not act in ways which might lead people to think they are untrustworthy. Thus a nurse who steals from people or is violent towards them, even when off duty, could not be said to be 'upholding the reputation of their profession'. This is because, a member of the public might find it difficult to trust a nurse who has a reputation for stealing, or feel safe with a nurse who has a reputation for having a short fuse. And it is crucial that patients feel they can trust nurses and feel safe when in their care.

These professional obligations have, at least in part, their moral foundations in principles of beneficence, non-maleficence and autonomy. Thus for example, it is necessary that patients trust nurses so that they will cooperate in treatment regimes and give relevant information to aid diagnosis and so on (family history of the relevant disorder, for example).

5. *Themselves?* A question mark is placed here due to unclarity surrounding what could be meant by such an obligation. Minimally, it denotes an obligation to be physically and mentally fit enough to perform one's professional duties. But construed in such a way it suggests that this obligation only holds because it is instrumental to the well-being of patients; that one is only obliged to stay fit and healthy so that others may benefit from one's state of health. Construed differently,

it may be held that one owes it to oneself to have a minimally decent standard of living with sufficient material comforts.

6. *Their dependents.* It is a view widely held among nurses and others of course that they have moral obligations to their dependents; and, further, that these are weightier than obligations to strangers. Again, the moral foundations of such obligations appear to be the principles of beneficence and non-maleficence. The relevance of beneficence here seems self-evident: one is under an obligation to act in ways which will benefit one's dependents.

With respect to non-maleficence, suppose one loses one's position as a consequence of drawing attention to poor standards of patient care. This may result in being unable to provide basic necessities for one's dependents, and it may be concluded by some nurses that they should keep quiet about their concerns (see e.g., Tadd, 1991; Hunt, 1994b; Dooley and McCarthy, 2005).

7. *Their employers.* Curtin and Flaherty (1982, p. 154) suggest that these are twofold. First, to practise as a competent professional; that is, to practise in accordance with the standards set out by the nurse's professional body – the NMC of course. Second, to be involved in the management of the institution to some degree. Curtin and Flaherty point out that some nurses explicitly have such a role – for example, nurse managers. But other nurses have such a role only implicitly, by their day-to-day decision-making; for example, concerning how best to use resources such as linen, sterile dressings, and so forth. One might usefully add a third obligation which nurses may plausibly be said to be bound by; namely, an obligation not to use health care resources wastefully. The code itself refers to obligations to 'inform any employers you work for if your fitness to practise is impaired or called into question' (NMC, 2008).

In the case of item 7 above, it seems reasonable to regard all three of these obligations as professional obligations; but what is their moral foundation?

Recall the claim referred to earlier that work for health is a moral endeavour – it involves working to promote a good; the good of restoring health or fostering autonomy. These considerations remind us that the moral foundation of health care work involves (at least) the principle of beneficence. It is the case that health care should result in good for patients (even if on occasion it does not). Also, the principle of non-maleficence is of central importance. The very least one would expect of work for health is that it does not result in harm to patients.

The benefits they obtain should outweigh any harms they may suffer (say, in undergoing surgery).

So, presumably, the point of health care institutions is to work for health, and to make possible the conditions under which nurses (and others) can work to benefit others – where they can carry out the obligations generated by the principle of beneficence. This suggests that nurses' obligations to their employers (and colleagues) and to the institutions in which they work, are only legitimate obligations in so far as they contribute to the general aim of making people well. So, although nurses are under an obligation not to squander health care resources, they are not under an obligation to be so frugal with health care resources that patient care suffers. In other words, the obligations nurses have towards their employers should not be permitted to overshadow the more fundamental obligations of the nurse; these being directed towards the patient. This point is worth labouring a little since the overall aim of the nurse's obligations to her employers can be lost sight of. It can seem that being frugal with resources – an obligation to the nurse's employers – can outweigh an obligation to benefit patient. But it should be clear that the obligations to patients are more fundamental since the obligations to employers and institutions only exist because of the obligations to patients. This ordering of the obligations of nurses seems, in fact, to be required by the NMC (2008) since, as we have seen, it states a duty to 'Make the care of people your first concern, treating them as individuals and respecting their dignity'.

Do nurses undertake supererogatory acts? Five nurse case examples

Having offered a rough but sufficiently sharp criterion of what constitutes a supererogatory act, and having identified the parties towards whom nurses can be said to have obligations, it can now be asked whether nurses do, in fact, undertake supererogatory acts. As we will see, it is evident that some nurses, at least, do perform actions which qualify as supererogatory. But, it is doubtful to claim that *all* nurses, merely by virtue of being members of the nursing profession, are routinely called upon to perform such acts, and to respond to that call. The case examples we consider now, though, do seem to describe situations in which the nurses act in ways which qualify as supererogatory. Moreover, they are not rare kinds of situations.

Consider the following five scenarios:

1. A ward manager, Jim Smith, in mental health nursing is coming towards the end of a difficult shift. The work has been particularly hard today, not least due to there being two new staff members who, through no fault of their own, have needed close supervision. Further, there have been two patients admitted to the ward during the shift, and these admissions proved to be more complex than is usual. A third patient is expected to be admitted at 3.30 p.m., and Jim is due to complete his shift at 3.00 p.m., having begun at 7.00 a.m.

At 2.30 p.m., Jim is informed that his colleague, June Brown, who is due to take charge of the ward at 3.00 p.m. is too ill to come into work. Jim's line manager asks him to work 'an extra hour' whilst he tries to arrange to cover Jim's ward. Jim has arranged to collect his children from school at 3.30 p.m. and it is too late to arrange for someone else to meet them. In any event, why should he even consider doing this?

Jim refuses to stay beyond 3.00 p.m. – though he feels guilty about this. A few minutes later, Jim's senior manager rings again. He sounds desperate and informs Jim that there is absolutely no means of covering Jim's ward between 3.00 and 4.00 p.m. Could Jim please reconsider? Think of the overtime payment he would receive. Jim now capitulates: not due to financial considerations, one hour's overtime is very little anyway, but he feels that he cannot leave the ward without knowing that cover has been confirmed; this would leave the new staff members in a vulnerable position, and the patients on the ward are likely to be affected too. Of course, the situation is made more complicated by the fact that a further patient is expected at 3.30 p.m.

What Jim has to do now though, and quickly, is to try to arrange for someone to collect his children. Fortunately, his partner is able to go to collect the children, despite the short notice. She is not happy about this change of arrangements, however, and she makes this clear to Jim. They had agreed that she would have that afternoon completely free so that she could complete an assignment for a course which she is studying.

As promised by Jim's manager, a replacement is found by 4.00 p.m. In spite of this, Jim does not eventually leave the ward until almost 4.30. His replacement is not familiar with the patients on the ward, and the patient due for admission at 3.30 arrived instead at 4.00 p.m. Jim felt obliged to stay at least until the initial disruption caused by a noisy new patient had subsided a little, and until his replacement had been given a very basic guide to what had been happening on the ward that day, and what to look out for during the next shift.

2. The second scenario arises in a busy accident and emergency unit. A patient with a superficial head wound and various other bumps, bruises and grazes enters the unit and asks to receive attention. He is asked to sit down and informed that he will be attended to as soon as possible. It is evident that the patient has been drinking. He becomes tired of waiting and exhibits extremely aggressive behaviour. He threatens to attack another patient sitting nearby. A nurse, Ann Baird, asks the violent patient either to leave the unit or to be more patient. The patient then physically assaults the nurse with a blow to the face. A struggle ensues. Whilst one nurse calls hospital security staff, others try to free Ann Baird from the grip of the patient; they too receive some kicks and blows from the patient. Eventually, he is overpowered and the police remove him from the unit. (Of course the problem of violence against NHS staff is growing problem; see BBC, 13/2/08; and BBC, 8/7/03.)

3. An alternative scenario involving a risk of violence to a nurse is the following. David Jones works in a community home, and six persons with quite serious learning difficulties live in the home. One of the residents, Jamie, has poor standards of personal hygiene. Further, Jamie resolutely refuses to have a bath, or even a wash. If efforts are made to press Jamie into having a wash, he becomes extremely aggressive. Over the years, a number of behaviour programmes have been attempted to change Jamie's attitude to washing but none has succeeded. Jamie's personal hygiene has deteriorated to such an extent that he now looks dirty and smells of stale perspiration. David, other staff members and residents feel that efforts should be made to persuade Jamie to have a wash, but he simply refuses. Staff members and residents alike are not sure what to do about the situation. Some staff members argue that if it is Jamie's decision not to wash, then this should be respected. Other staff, and the other five residents, are less sure of this. They think Jamie should be coerced into having a wash. Eventually, it is decided that David should try to pressurize Jamie into having a wash, even though this is against Jamie's wishes. David is apprehensive about taking on this task as he knows that Jamie could become aggressive and he is a strong and powerful young man. In spite of this, David attempts to implement the course of action agreed upon by the staff group and the other five residents.

4. Recently, it was reported that a nurse in the United Kingdom had died as a result of contracting HIV during the course of her nursing

duties (BBC, 2/12/08). And in their discussion of supererogation, Beauchamp and Childress refer to obligations to care for patients with dangerous, transmissible diseases, such as SARS (severe acute respiratory syndrome; 2009, p. 50)). They query whether such obligations may legitimately be demanded of health care professionals, or whether undertaking such work should, more properly, be 'optional' (2009, p. 50; see also Johnstone, 1999, p. 402). Consider, then, the following case example.

Sue is employed in a special unit for the care of persons who are HIV-positive. As is well documented, there is only a very small risk of transmission of the virus to health care workers via, for example, needle stick injuries. In fact, the risk of acquiring HIV from a needle stick injury is believed to be around 0.3 per cent (see e.g., Schecter, 1992, p. 223).) Sue occasionally thinks about the risks of acquiring the virus during the course of her work, but she does not dwell on this for too long. Her partner, though, does harbour concerns about the risk of transmission and, from time to time, the fact that in the eyes of her partner Sue deliberately exposes herself to this risk, is a cause of tension between them.

5. Simon is a Community Psychiatric Nurse and has an extremely heavy and diverse case-load. At the last count, he found that he has responsibility for over 40 extremely vulnerable patients in addition to providing assessments for a local GP practice and managing a medication clinic. Many of Simon's patients are in need of closer supervision than he can provide – there are only 24 hours in a day. Frequently, Simon finds that he works over 12 hours a day. For at least three of those hours he is generally not paid, since his managers refuse to pay overtime for them. He has since stopped even trying to claim payments for any extra hours he works. Simon has complained bitterly to his managers that he is overworked, and that his case-load is far too big. Recently, a patient of Simon physically assaulted a complete stranger; the assault, it seems, was attributable to a deterioration in the mental health of the patient. She had been diagnosed as suffering from schizophrenia and had not taken medication prescribed for her – she had not turned up for the last two appointments at which she would be given medication by injection. Simon felt responsible in some way for the assault on the stranger, and for the deterioration in the mental health of his patient. With a smaller case-load, he felt sure he would have been better able to monitor his patient's mental health and thus prevent the harms suffered both by his patient and by the stranger.

Simon feels that his work dominates so much of his life that he has little time for interests outside of work. When he does get home he feels too exhausted to do anything other than watch TV and drink alcohol. He recognizes that his lifestyle is stressful and extremely unhealthy, and feels exasperated that there seems to be no end in sight to his present situation.

Consider the predicament of the nurses in the above examples. Recall that following Beauchamp and Childress we defined supererogatory acts as those which are optional, are for the benefit of others, and go beyond what would be expected by ordinary moral standards, for example by virtue of the extent to which they expose the actor to significant risk of harm (2009, p. 48).

In case one, Jim Smith is in a situation which raises conflicts of obligations to colleagues, patients, his immediate managers at the hospital, his dependents and partner, and, perhaps also, to himself. In short, the obligations to patients, colleagues and hospital managers seem to conflict with his obligations to his family and to himself. Jim ultimately gives greater weight to the obligations to the first groups just mentioned than to the obligations to his family and himself. His actions, it seems, are for the benefit of others – specifically his patient and his colleagues, even though they have at least two undesirable consequences: they deprive him of the pleasure of collecting his children, and they cause strain in the relationship between Jim and his partner. Each of these consequences, especially the second perhaps, can be described as harms which Jim undergoes; harms which result from actions which are intended to benefit others. Thus it looks like Jim's actions qualify as supererogatory.

In the second case example, it seems that Ann Baird's actions also qualify as supererogatory if she recognizes that it is likely that the patient will become aggressive. Her action is for the benefit of others – not least the patient himself – but is one which exposes her to risk of significant harm. The same can be said of the colleagues who go to Ann's aid: they are exposing themselves to risk of harm for the benefit of others – in this case, Ann and other patients. In this incident, the obligations to others are apparently given greater weight by the nurses involved than the obligations to themselves.

With regard to the scenario involving David Jones and Jamie, here again it seems that David's action can be classed as a supererogatory action. He is exposing himself to risk of physical harms for the benefit of others – for example, possibly Jamie, and certainly the other staff and residents. In this case example, David places obligations to others above those to himself.

In the fourth example, it was suggested that Sue exposes herself to risk of infection during the course of her work. It should be repeated that the actual probability of acquiring HIV during the course of her normal duties is quite low (Schecter, 1992). But of course, although the probability of infection may in fact be extremely low, the level of potential harm is extremely high: Sue is exposed to a small risk of acquiring a life-threatening infection (recall the actual case referred to earlier in which the nurse actually loses her life as a result of acquiring HIV at work). If the risk of infection were low, and the potential hazard not especially harmful, then it seems unlikely that Sue's role could be described as one which involves the undertaking of supererogatory actions. But, as we have seen, the magnitude of harm to which Sue exposes herself, for the benefit of others, is very great indeed. Hence, it does not seem implausible to claim that her role involves the undertaking of supererogatory actions.

The fifth example offered involved Simon, the Community Psychiatric Nurse. Due to an unreasonably heavy workload, he is unable to fulfil quite basic obligations to himself. Specifically, he finds it impossible to carve out any leisure time. This means that he cannot meet the obligations to himself in either of the two senses identified earlier: his work commitments prevent him from engaging in a life beyond work; and the same commitments seem to be driving him to a state of psychological ill health. Hence, he cannot meet the obligations to himself even when these are construed instrumentally.

Since, as in the previous examples, Simon's actions are motivated by an intention to benefit his clients, it seems again that his actions qualify as supererogatory acts.

It may be argued that none of the nurses we have considered act in ways which are describable as supererogatory. The reason why, it may be said, is that it is simply part of the nurse's role – the nurse's station, so to speak – to undertake the kinds of actions described in the examples just offered. Since nurses are paid for their work, it may be added, their actions cannot be described as supererogatory. This is because the 'voluntariness' of the actions is not present. It is not present because nurses are supposed to care for people and that is all that the nurses in our examples are doing.

There are at least two ways of responding to such an argument. The first simply exploits the conclusion reached in Chapter 1, to the effect that there is a necessary relationship between ethics and nursing practice. Since the actions of the nurses in our examples satisfy the criterion for classification as actions with a moral aspect to them, the fact that the nurses are paid for their actions does not affect the claim that they are actions with a moral dimension to them.

It might also be pointed out that in the cases we described, the intentions of the nurses are uniformly to act in ways which benefit their patients and which expose themselves to certain harms. The acts are optional because although nurses are required to acts in ways which benefit others they are not required to do so to the extent that their own interests are harmed. In the examples given that is just what is taking place. These considerations themselves seem to suggest that their actions meet the criterion of supererogatory acts put forward by Beauchamp and Childress (2009, p. 48) and described above. This is the case even if they receive payment for such actions.

A different strategy to query whether the nurses described in our case examples are undertaking supererogatory actions is to focus, not on the fact that nurses are paid for their work, but, as mentioned, to claim it is part of the 'station' of the nurse to act as the nurses described above have acted. An argument such as this might exploit the points we have made about nursing being inherently a moral enterprise. Thus, although it may be the case that by ordinary moral standards obligations of beneficence to others do not figure prominently, they are an intrinsic part of the nursing role. This is of course made plain in the code of conduct: 'you must work with others to protect *and promote* the health and wellbeing of those in your care' (NMC, 2008). Thus, it may be claimed, extraordinary moral standards are expected of those of who enter the nursing profession. So, nurses such as Simon, Ann and Jim are not acting in ways which are supererogatory, relative to the moral standards required in nursing practice.

If one were to accept this conclusion it would follow that the nurses we describe should continue to place obligations to others above those to themselves and their loved ones, and hence to harm themselves in order to benefit others. I take it that this is not an acceptable conclusion. Working conditions should be such that it is possible for nurses to contribute fully to patient care without routinely jeopardizing their own health. To say this, of course, is not to say that in some circumstances of care a nurse might choose to do something that will expose her to high risk of harm and do so for the benefit of others. Perhaps a nurse who works in an area affected by plague, famine or war would count as such a nurse. So it seems plausible to claim a distinction within nursing roles which recognizes that some 'role obligations' are obligatory, they are indeed part of the nurses station. But at the same time there are some actions conducted by some nurses, in their role as a nurse, which exceed these ordinary role obligations and merit the title of supererogatory acts.

Beauchamp and Childress suggest a distinction can be drawn between 'ordinary role obligations and extraordinary self-imposed standards' (2009, p. 48). It is plausible to think that acts motivated by extraordinary self-imposed standards qualify as supererogatory – even given the 'higher than ordinary' moral standards expected in the context of nursing. So, the nurses in our five examples, it may be said, have extraordinarily high self-imposed standards. If this is true, it does not follow that it is reasonable to expect all nurses to be bound by such exacting standards.

Thus, consider a nurse who is placed in a situation such as that faced by Jim, but who responds differently. Suppose this nurse simply refuses to stay on beyond her official span of duty (it can be imagined that she has stayed on previous occasions but has decided that enough is enough). It can reasonably be supposed that the most one's ordinary role obligations require one to do is to work the number of hours one is contracted to work – perhaps with a small degree of flexibility on the part of the nurse. The standards which Jim imposes upon himself amount to extraordinary standards since, as seen above, they place obligations to promote the health of patients above those to his own family, and thus to his own well-being.

A parallel claim can be made in relation to Simon: his actions seem to exceed ordinary role obligations. Perhaps the actions of David fall into this category also. The reason is that he is exposing himself to significant risk of significant physical harm, and is doing so for the benefit of other parties (supposedly, including Jamie). It is implausible to claim that exposing oneself to high risk of serious physical injury could be regarded as an ordinary role obligation. This is certainly in the context of nursing, even if it is not true for example of members of the armed forces. Hence, it is plausible to uphold the claim that the nurses in the example given above do act in ways which qualify as supererogatory. More importantly, perhaps, it is also true that there can be no expectation that such harmful role obligations become expected as the norm.

Now, it may be said of Simon, and perhaps also of Jim, that he should simply try harder to obtain more support; that is, it may be said that there are simply insufficient levels of staff to meet the demand placed upon the mental health services in his area. To that

extent, it can be seen that Simon's predicament is significantly different from that of Sue. Although it has been claimed that both Simon
and Sue engage in supererogatory actions, Sue is at least able to meet
the needs of her patients without working longer hours than she is
paid to do. She, at least, has opportunities to meet obligations to herself, to her dependents (if any) and to her partner. Simon, it seems, is
deprived of such opportunities. Perhaps also, the same may be said to
a lesser extent of Jim.

A more philosophical point would be to emphasize some of the points
made in Chapter 3 and in the previous chapter, where we appealed to
the idea of a life plan. Occupational roles which so dominate the life
of a person to the extent that they are unable to do anything outside
of their working role, unless part of a person's life plan, so obstruct
the pursuance of a life plan that they can be viewed as unacceptably
demanding. Hence there can be no requirement for nurses to tolerate
what is intolerable. So whilst it is of course obligatory to 'make the
care of people your first concern' and 'to provide a high standard of
practice and care at all times' (NMC, 2008) it cannot be considered
obligatory for nurses routinely to jeopardize their own prospects for a
flourishing, autonomous life. This is an important point since it gives a
rough criterion for distinguishing ordinary role and extraordinary role
obligations. The significance of this is that whilst it is obligatory to perform acts which are part of their ordinary role obligations, there is no
similar obligation routinely to perform acts which are extraordinary.
These are acts which benefit others but expose the actor to significant
risk of harm. When it comes to spelling out what counts as 'significant
harm' there are obvious ones such as are presented by caring for violent patients, or exposing oneself to risk of infection of serious diseases
such as HIV. But it is less obvious to explain the way in which the
kinds of working patterns described, especially in the case of Simon,
qualify as seriously harmful. This is because the harms concern a pattern of behaviour as opposed to exposure to an obvious danger, such
as HIV infection or assault. But we can exploit the point above regarding pursuance of a 'life plan' to articulate the way in which the kinds of
patterns of behaviours undertaken by Simon and Jim are unacceptable.
This is because these working patterns seriously impugn their prospects
of pursuing an autonomously chosen life plan. Work so dominates
their life that they lack time to pursue other things which are important to them, important in terms of their leading a good life according
to their conception of what that consists in – be it being a good 'family
man' as Jim tries to be, or a person who has time for things other than

work, as Simon tries to be. Of course, it may be that being perpetually available to help others is part of a person's conception of what is a good life for them – part of their life plan. So, Simon's lengthy working hours would not be such a problem for such a person. When people refer to 'moral saints' (see Beauchamp and Childress, 2009, p. 53) it is likely that this is the kind of person they have in mind. It is someone for whom the most important thing in life is helping others. What is plain, though, is that such people are exceptional. Their behaviours, by definition, cannot be held up as what should routinely be expected of nurses. This is because, obviously, the quality of being saintlike is rare, so it is absurd to expect this to be displayed routinely by nurses (or any other professional group). This discussion illustrates, then, that the kinds of lifestyle into which Simon has been pressed is not is a life-style which it is acceptable to expect him to put up with simply because he is a nurse, and a central part of nursing role is to help others. The obligations that one takes on in becoming a nurse are not unlimited. When seeking to fulfil one's obligations is incompatible with leading a good, rounded, life one is placed in an impossible situation and should not think it is something one has to learn to live with.

Conclusion

In this final chapter, then, we have seen how the principles help to structure thinking about a very abstract idea, that of supererogatory acts. In contrast to the conclusion to the corresponding chapter in the first edition of this book, it has been possible to be a bit more con-clusive. For, by exploiting the idea of a life plan, in conjunction with the principles, it has been possible to explain why it is not coherent to expect the kinds of working patterns endured by Simon, for example in our discussion, to be accepted routinely by nurses. Some people exhibit saintlike behaviour which is, by definition *exceptional, untypical*, so this cannot be required or even routinely expected of nursing staff.

Appendix:
NMC Code of
Conduct (2008)

The Code
Standards of conduct, performance and ethics for nurses and midwives

The people in your care must be able to trust you with their health and well-being. To justify that trust, you must

- make the care of people your first concern, treating them as individuals and respecting their dignity

- work with others to protect and promote the health and wellbeing of those in your care, their families and carers, and the wider community

- provide a high standard of practice and care at all times

- be open and honest, act with integrity and uphold the reputation of your profession

As a professional, you are personally accountable for actions and omissions in your practice and must always be able to justify your decisions.

You must always act lawfully, whether those laws relate to your professional practice or personal life.

Failure to comply with this Code may bring your fitness to practise into question and endanger your registration.

This Code should be considered together with the Nursing and Midwifery Council's rules, standards, guidance and advice available from www.nmc-uk.org.

Make the care of people your first concern, treating them as individuals and respecting their dignity

Treat people as individuals

- You must treat people as individuals and respect their dignity
- You must not discriminate in any way against those in your care
- You must treat people kindly and considerately
- You must act as an advocate for those in your care, helping them to access relevant health and social care, information and support

Respect people's confidentiality

- You must respect people's right to confidentiality
- You must ensure people are informed about how and why information is shared by those who will be providing their care
- You must disclose information if you believe someone may be at risk of harm, in line with the law of the country in which you are practising

Collaborate with those in your care

- You must listen to the people in your care and respond to their concerns and preferences
- You must support people in caring for themselves to improve and maintain their health
- You must recognise and respect the contribution that people make to their own care and wellbeing
- You must make arrangements to meet people's language and communication needs

- You must share with people, in a way they can understand, the information they want or need to know about their health

Ensure you gain consent

- You must ensure that you gain consent before you begin any treatment or care
- You must respect and support people's rights to accept or decline treatment and care
- You must uphold people's rights to be fully involved in decisions about their care
- You must be aware of the legislation regarding mental capacity, ensuring that people who lack capacity remain at the centre of decision making and are fully safeguarded
- You must be able to demonstrate that you have acted in someone's best interests if you have provided care in an emergency

Maintain clear professional boundaries

- You must refuse any gifts, favours or hospitality that might be interpreted as an attempt to gain preferential treatment
- You must not ask for or accept loans from anyone in your care or anyone close to them
- You must establish and actively maintain clear sexual boundaries at all times with people in your care, their families and carers

Work with others to protect and promote the health and wellbeing of those in your care, their families and carers, and the wider community

Share information with your colleagues

- You must keep your colleagues informed when you are sharing the care of others
- You must work with colleagues to monitor the quality of your work and maintain the safety of those in your care
- You must facilitate students and others to develop their competence

Work effectively as part of a team

- You must work cooperatively within teams and respect the skills, expertise and contributions of your colleagues
- You must be willing to share your skills and experience for the benefit of your colleagues
- You must consult and take advice from colleagues when appropriate
- You must treat your colleagues fairly and without discrimination
- You must make a referral to another practitioner when it is in the best interests of someone in your care

Delegate effectively

- You must establish that anyone you delegate to is able to carry out your instructions
- You must confirm that the outcome of any delegated task meets required standards
- You must make sure that everyone you are responsible for is supervised and supported

Manage risk

- You must act without delay if you believe that you, a colleague or anyone else may be putting someone at risk
- You must inform someone in authority if you experience problems that prevent you working within this Code or other nationally agreed standards
- You must report your concerns in writing if problems in the environment of care are putting people at risk

Provide a high standard of practice and care at all times

Use the best available evidence

- You must deliver care based on the best available evidence or best practice.

- You must ensure any advice you give is evidence based if you are suggesting healthcare products or services

- You must ensure that the use of complementary or alternative therapies is safe and in the best interests of those in your care

Keep your skills and knowledge up to date

- You must have the knowledge and skills for safe and effective practice when working without direct supervision

- You must recognise and work within the limits of your competence

- You must keep your knowledge and skills up to date throughout your working life

- You must take part in appropriate learning and practice activities that maintain and develop your competence and performance

Keep clear and accurate records

- You must keep clear and accurate records of the discussions you have, the assessments you make, the treatment and medicines you give and how effective these have been

- You must complete records as soon as possible after an event has occurred

- You must not tamper with original records in any way

- You must ensure any entries you make in someone's paper records are clearly and legibly signed, dated and timed

- You must ensure any entries you make in someone's electronic records are clearly, attributable to you

- You must ensure all records are kept confidentially and securely

Be open and honest, act with integrity and uphold the reputation of your profession

Act with integrity

- You must demonstrate a personal and professional commitment to equality and diversity

- You must adhere to the laws of the country in which you are practising
- You must inform the NMC if you have been cautioned, charged or found guilty of a criminal offence
- You must inform any employers you work for if your fitness to practise is impaired or is called into question

Deal with problems

- You must give a constructive and honest response to anyone who complains about the care they have received
- You must not allow someone's complaint to prejudice the care you provide for them
- You must act immediately to put matters right if someone in your care has suffered harm for any reason
- You must explain fully and promptly to the person affected what has happened and the likely effects
- You must cooperate with internal and external investigations

Be impartial

- You must not abuse your privileged position for your own ends
- You must ensure that your professional judgment is not influenced by any commercial Considerations

Uphold the reputation of your profession

- You must not use your professional status to promote causes that are not related to health
- You must cooperate with the media only when you can confidently protect the confidential information and dignity of those in your care
- You must uphold the reputation of your profession at all times

Information about indemnity insurance

The NMC recommends that a registered nurse, midwife or specialist community public health nurse, in advising, treating and caring for patients/clients, has professional indemnity insurance. This is in the interests of clients, patients and registrants in the event of claims of professional negligence.

Whilst employers have vicarious liability for the negligent acts and/or omissions of their employees, such cover does not normally extend to activities undertaken outside the registrant's employment. Independent practice would not be covered by vicarious liability. It is the individual registrant's responsibility to establish their insurance status and take appropriate action.

In situations where an employer does not have vicarious liability, the NMC recommends that registrants obtain adequate professional indemnity insurance. If unable to secure professional indemnity insurance, a registrant will need to demonstrate that all their clients/patients are fully informed of this fact and the implications this might have in the event of a claim for professional negligence.

Contact

Nursing & Midwifery Council
23 Portland Place
London W1B 1PZ

020 7333 9333
advice@nmc-uk.org
www.nmc-uk.org

Healthcare professionals have a shared set of values, which find their expression in this Code for nurses and midwives. These values are also reflected in the different codes of each of the UK's healthcare regulators. This Code was approved by the NMC's Council on 6 December 2007 for implementation on 1 May 2008.

Available from: http://www.nmc-uk.org/aArticle.aspx?ArticleID=3056

Bibliography

Agar, N. (2004), *Liberal Eugenics, in Defence of Human Enhancement* (Oxford: Blackwell).

Alderson, P. (1990), *Choosing for Children* (Oxford: Oxford University Press).

Alderson, P. (1992), 'Defining ethics in nursing practice', *Nursing Standard* 6, pp. 33–5.

Alderson, P. (2001), 'Down's syndrome: cost, quality and value of life', *Social Sciences and Medicine* 53, pp. 627–38.

Aristotle, *Nichomachean Ethics* (1955), (trans.), Thompson, J. A. K. (Harmondsworth: Penguin).

Aristotle, 'Metaphysics', in Ackrill, J. L. (ed.) (1987), *A New Aristotle Reader* (Oxford: Oxford University Press) pp. 255–360.

Armstrong, A. E. (2007), *Nursing Ethics, a Virtue-Based Approach* (Basingstoke: Palgrave).

Aspis, S. and Souza, A. 'People with Down's syndrome disrupt screening conference', published 30/5/03 (available at: http://www.worldenable.net/rights/adhoc2meetbulletin05.htm) accessed 5/8/08.

Baier, A. C. (1985), 'What women want in a moral theory', in Larrabee (ed.) 1993, pp. 19–32.

Bandman, E. L. and Bandman, B. (1990), *Nursing Ethics Through the Lifespan*, 2nd edn (London: Prentice-Hall).

Barker, J. (1995), *Local NHS Healthcare Purchasing and Prioritising from the Perspective of Bromley Residents* (Hayes: Bromley Health).

Barr, O. G. and McConkey, R. (2006), 'Supporting parents who have a child referred for genetic investigation: the contribution of health visitors', *Journal of Advanced Nursing* 2006 54(2), pp. 141–50.

BBC (1994), *Hypotheticals* (London: BBC Publications).

BBC, 'Mixed sex NHS still a problem', published 19/5/08 (available at: http://news.bbc.co.uk/1/hi/health/7408771.stm) accessed 20/5/08.

BBC, 'Urgent action on maternity units', published 20/5/08 (available at: http://news.bbc.co.uk/1/hi/wales/7411241.stm) accessed 21/5/08.

BBC, 'Inside the ethics committee', broadcast 28/8/07 (available at: www.bbc.co.uk/radio4/science/ethicscommittee_s3_tr1.shtml) accessed 16/1/08.

BBC, 'Mother dies after refusing blood' (Emma Gough case), published 5/11/07 (available at: http://news.bbc.co.uk/1/hi/england/shropshire/7078455.stm) accessed 21/11/08.

BBC, 'The ward smelt of diarrhoea', published 11/10/07 (available at: http://news.bbc.co.uk/1/hi/health/7038107.stm) accessed 21/11/08.

BBC, 'Care staff sedated him by 4.00 p.m.', published 27/11/07 (available at: http://news.bbc.co.uk/1/hi/health/7113559.stm) accessed 21/11/08.

BBC, 'Call to redirect cancer drug cash', published 29/11/07 (available at: http://news.bbc.co.uk/1/hi/health/7115540.stm) accessed 21/11/08.

BBC, 'Mental health nurses face attacks', published 13/2/08(available at: http://news.bbc.co.uk/1/hi/health/7241453.stm) accessed 6/8/08.

BBC, 'Attacks against NHS staff soar', published 8/7/03 (available at: http://news.bbc.co.uk/1/hi/health/3051090.stm) accessed 18/4/08.

BBC, 'Nurse contracted HIV from patient', published 12/2/08 (available at: http://news.bbc.co.uk/1/hi/england/london/7241951.stm) accessed 6/8/08.

BBC, 'No regrets for cancer sisters', published 15/1/08 (available at: http://news.bbc.co.uk/1/hi/england/south_yorkshire/7189404.stm) accessed 16/1/08.

Beauchamp, T. L. and Childress, J. F. (1989), *Principles of Biomedical Ethics*, 3rd edn (Oxford: Oxford University Press).

Beauchamp, T. L. and Childress, J. F. (1994), *Principles of Biomedical Ethics*, 4th edn (Oxford: Oxford University Press).

Beauchamp, T. L., and Childress J. F. (**2001**), *Principles of Biomedical Ethics*, 5th edn (Oxford Oxford University Press).

Beauchamp, T. L., and Childress, J. F. (2009), *Principles of Biomedical Ethics*, 6th edn (Oxford: Oxford University Press).

Begg, J. (2003), 'Twenty years ago, the first clues to the birth of a plague', NY Times (available at: http://www.nytimes.com/2001/06/03/weekinreview/03WORD.html?ex=1227330000&en=e9ff3187797e805b&ei=5070) accessed 4/12/07.

Benjamin, M. and Curtis, J. (1986), *Ethics in Nursing*, 2nd edn (Oxford: Oxford University Press).

Benjamin, M. and Curtis, J. (1992), *Ethics in Nursing*, 3rd edn (Oxford: Oxford University Press).

Benner, P. and Wrubel, J. (1989), *The Primacy of Caring, Stress and Coping in Health and Illness* (Menlo Park, California: Addison-Wesley).

Berghmans, R. and Widdershoven, G. (2007) 'Physician assisted dying in the Netherlands', EACME newsletter, 17, 24/8/07, pp.13–22 (available at: http://www.eacmeweb.com/newsletter/n17.htm) accessed 16/1/08.

Bloch, S. and Chodoff, P. (eds) (1981), *Psychiatric Ethics* (Oxford: Oxford University Press).

Bluglass, R. (1993), 'The case for supervision', *Nursing Times* 89(6), pp. 32–3.

Blum, L. (1988), 'Gilligan and Kohlberg: Implications for moral theory', in Larrabee (ed.) (1993), pp. 49–68.

BMA (2007), 'Decisions relating to cardiopulmonary resuscitation', Oct. 2007(available at: www.bma.org) accessed 16/1/08.

Bowden, P. (1997), *Caring: Gender-Sensitive Ethics* (London: Routledge).

Brabeck, M. (1983), 'Moral judgment: theory and research on differences between males and females', in Larrabee (ed.) (1993), pp. 33–48.

Brown, A. (1986), *Modern Political Philosophy* (Harmondsworth: Penguin).

Brown, J. M., Kitson, A. L. and McKnight, T. J. (1992), *Challenges in Caring* (London: Chapman & Hall).

Buchanan, A. E. and Brock, D. W. (1990), *Deciding for Others* (Cambridge: Cambridge University Press).

Buchanan, A. E., Brock, D. W., Daniels, N. and Wikler, D. (2000), *From Chance to Choice, Genetics and Justice* (Cambridge: Cambridge University Press).

Burnard, P. and Chapman, C. M. (1988), *Professional and Ethical Issues in Nursing* (Chichester: John Wiley).

Camus, A. (1955), *The Myth of Sisyphus* (Harmondsworth: Penguin).

Capuzzi, C. and Garland, M. (1990), 'The Oregon plan: increasing access to health care', *Nursing Outlook* Nov./Dec., pp. 260–86.

Card, C. (1990), 'Caring and evil', *Hypatia* 5(1), pp. 101–8.

Carr, B. (1987), *Metaphysics: an Introduction* (London: Macmillan).

Cash, K. (1990), 'Nursing models and the idea of nursing', *International Journal of Nursing Studies* 27 (3), pp. 249–56.

Chadwick, R. and Tadd, W. (1992), *Ethics and Nursing Practice* (London: Macmillan).

Clark, M. (1977), *Practical Nursing* (London: Balliere-Tindall).

Clouser, K. D. and Gert, B. (1990), 'A critique of principlism', *The Journal of Medicine and Philosophy* 15, pp. 219–36.

Cox, S. M. (2004), Human genetics, ethics and disability, in Storch, J. L., Rodney, P. and Starzomski, R. (eds) (2004) *Towards a Moral Horizon, Nursing Ethics for Leadership and Practice* (Toronto: Pearson), pp.378–95.

Culver, C. M. and Gert, B. (1982), *Philosophy in Medicine* (New York: Oxford University Press).

Curtin, L. and Flaherty, M. J. (1982), *Nursing Ethics: Theories and Pragmatics* (London: Prentice Hall).

Dancy, J. and Sosa, E. (1992), *A Companion to Epistemology* (Oxford: Blackwell).

Daniels, N. (1985), *Just Health Care* (Cambridge: Cambridge University Press).

Davis, A. J., Tschudin, V., and de Raeve, L. (eds) (2006), *Essentials of Teaching and Learning in Nursing Ethics* (London: Churchill Livingstone).

Department of Health (1991), *The Patient's Charter* (London: HMSO).

Department of Health (1993), 'Guidance for staff on relations with the public and the media' (London: DoH).

Department of Health (2006), Consultation on core principles...' (London: DoH).

Department of Health (2007), 'Human rights in healthcare – a framework for local action' (London: DoH).

De Raeve, L. (2002), 'Trust and trustworthiness in the nurse-patient relationship', *Nursing Philosophy* 3(2), 152–62.

Dickenson, D. (1994), 'Nurse time as a scarce health care resource', in Hunt (ed.) (1994a), pp. 207–17.

Dock, L. L. (1900), 'Ethics, or a code of ethics?' in Dock L. L., *Short Papers on Nursing Subjects* (New York: Longeway).

Dooley, D. and McCarthy, J. (2005), *Nursing Ethics, Irish Cases and Concerns* (Dublin: Gill & MacMillan).

Downie, R. S. and Calman, K. C. (1987), *Healthy Respect* (London: Faber & Faber).

Dworkin, G. (1971), 'Paternalism', in Wasserstrom, R. (ed.) (1971), *Morality and the Law* (Belmont: Wadsworth), pp. 107–26.

Dworkin, G. (1988), *The Theory and Practice of Autonomy* (Cambridge: Cambridge University Press).

Dworkin, R. (1977), *Taking Rights Seriously* (London: Duckworth).

Edwards, S. D. (1990), *Relativism, Conceptual Schemes and Categorial Frameworks* (Aldershot: Avebury).

Edwards, S. D. (2001), *Philosophy of Nursing: an Introduction* (London: Palgrave).

Edwards, S. D. (2005), *Disability, Definition, Value & Identity* (Oxford: Radcliffe).

Edwards, S. D. (2006), 'A principle-based approach to nursing ethics', in Davis, Tschudin, and de Raeve (eds), pp. 55–66.

Edwards, S. D. (2007), 'The nurse-patient relationship: a "principles plus care" account', in Ashcroft, R. E., Dawson, A., Draper, H. and McMillan, J. R. (eds), *Principles of Health Care Ethics,* 2nd edn(Chichester: Wiley) pp. 365–70.

Fairbairn, G. J. (1995), *Contemplating Suicide* (London: Routledge).

Faulder, C. (1985), *Whose Body is it?* (London: Virago).

Feyerabend, P. (1975), *Against Method* (London: Verso).

Frankena, W. J. (1973), *Ethics* (London: Prentice-Hall).

'Free to leave at any time', *Open Mind*, no. 52, pp. 7–10.

Frey, R. G. (1983), *Rights, Killing and Suffering* (Oxford: Blackwell).

Friedman, M. (1987), 'Beyond caring: the de-moralisation of gender', in Larrabee (ed.) (1993), pp. 258–73.

Fry, S. (1989), 'The role of caring in a theory of nursing ethics', *Hypatia* 4(2), pp. 88–103

Fuller, S. (1988), *Social Epistemology* (Bloomington: Indiana University Press).

Gastmans, C. (2006), 'The care perspective in healthcare ethics', in Davis, Tschudin and de Raeve (eds), pp.135–48.

'The Gay plague' (1982) in *NY Magazine*, published September 1982 (extracts available at: http://www.nytimes.com/2001/06/03/weekinreview/03WORD. html?ex=1227330000&en=e9ff3187797e805b&ei=5070) accessed 4/12/07.

Gilligan, C. (1982), *In a Different Voice* (Cambridge, MA: Harvard University Press).

Gilligan, C. (1986), 'Reply to critics', in Larrabee (ed.) (1993), pp. 207–14.

Gillon, R. (1985), *Philosophical Medical Ethics* (Chichester: John Wiley). [year is 1986 in Ch 3]

Gillon R. (2003) 'Ethics needs principles', *Journal of Medical Ethics* 29, pp. 307–12.

Gillon, R. (ed.) (1994), *Principles of Health Care Ethics* (Chichester: John Wiley).

Glover, J. (1977), *Causing Death and Saving Lives* (Harmondsworth: Penguin).

Green, R. (1976), 'Health care and justice in contract theory perspective', in Veatch, R. and Branson, R. (eds) (1976), *Ethics and Health Policy* (Cambridge, MA: Ballinger), pp. 111–26.

Hampshire, S. (ed.) (1978), *Public and Private Morality* (Cambridge: Cambridge University Press).

Hanfling, O. (1972), *Kant's Copernican Revolution* (Milton Keynes: Open University Press).

Hanford, L. (1994), 'Nursing and the concept of care', in Hunt (ed.) (1994a), pp. 181–97.

Hare, R. M. (1981), *Moral Thinking* (Oxford: Oxford University Press).

Harris, J. (1985), *The Value of Life* (London: Routledge).

Hewitt, J. and Edwards, S. D. (2006), Moral perspectives on the prevention of suicide in mental health settings', *Journal of Psychiatric and Mental Health Nursing* 13, pp. 665–72..

Honderich, T. and Burnyeat, M. (eds) (1979), *Philosophy as It Is* (Harmondsworth: Pelican).

Houlihan, G. D. (2000), The nurses' power to detain informal psychiatric patients, a review of the statutory and common law provisions in England and Wales', *Journal of Advanced Nursing* 32(4), pp. 864–70.

Human Tissue Act (2004), Great Britain, Her Majesty's Stationary Office (HMSO).

Hunt, G. (ed.) (1994a), *Ethical Issues in Nursing* (London: Routledge).

Hunt, G. (ed.) (1994b), *Whistleblowing in the Health Service* (London: Edward Arnold).

Hursthouse, R. (1999), *On Virtue Ethics* (Oxford: Oxford University Press).

Hussey, T. (1990), 'Nursing ethics and project 2000', *Journal of Advanced Nursing* 15, pp. 1377–82.

Johnstone, M. J. (1989), *Bioethics: a Nursing Perspective* (London: Bailliere-Tindall).

Johnstone, M. J. (1999), *Bioethics: a Nursing Perspective*, 3rd edn (London: Bailliere-Tindall).

Kant, I. [1785 (1948)], 'Groundwork of the metaphysic of morals', in Paton, H. A. (trans.), The Moral Law (London: Hutchinson).

Kim, J. (1976), 'Events as property exemplifications', in Brand, M. and Walton, D. (eds), *Action Theory* (Dordrecht: Reidel), pp. 158–77.

Kittay, E. and Meyers, D. (eds) (1987), *Women and Moral Theory* (New Jersey: Rowman & Littlefield).

Kleinberg, S. S. (1991), *Politics and Philosophy* (Oxford: Blackwell).

Kohlberg, L. (1981), *The Philosophy of Moral Development* (San Francisco: Harper & Row).

Korenromp, M. J., Page-Christaens, G. C. M. L., van den Bout, J. (et al.) (2007), 'A prospective study on parental coping after termination of pregnancy for fetal anomalies', *Prenatal Diagnosis* 27(8), p. 709.

Kuhn, T. S. (1962), *The Structure of Scientific Revolutions* (Chicago: Chicago University Press).

Kymlicka, W. (1990), *Contemporary Political Philosophy* (Oxford: Oxford University Press).

Kuhse, H. and Singer, P. (1985), *Should the Baby Live?* (Oxford: Oxford University Press).

Larrabee, M. J. (ed.) (1993), *An Ethic of Care* (London: Routledge).

Leininger, M. M. (ed.) (1984), *Care: The Essence of Nursing and Health* (New York: Slack).

Little M. (1998), 'Care: from theory to orientation and back', *Journal of Medicine and Philosophy* 23, pp. 190–209.

Loach, E. (2003), 'The hardest thing I have ever done', published 31/5/03 (available at: http://www.guardian.co.uk/society/2003/may/31/health.lifeandhealth) accessed 5/8/08.

Loehy, E. H. (1991), 'Involving patients in DNR decisions', *Journal of Medical Ethics,* 17, pp. 156–60.

Lutzen, K. (1998), 'Subtle coercion in psychiatric practice', *Journal of Psychiatric and Mental Health Nursing 5*, pp. 101–7.

Lyons, D. (1965), *Forms and Limits of Utilitarianism* (Oxford: Clarendon Press).

Macdonald, C. (1989), *Mind-Body Identity Theories* (London: Routledge).

Maclean, A. (1993), *The Elimination of Morality* (London: Routledge).

Marquis, D. (1989), 'Why abortion is immoral', *Journal of Philosophy* LXXXVI(4), pp. 183–202.

Mason, J. K. and McCall Smith, R. A. (1994), *Law and Medical Ethics,* 4th edn (London: Butterworths).

McKenna, G. (1993), 'Caring is the essence of nursing practice', *British Journal of Nursing* 2(1), pp. 72–6.

Melia, K. (1989), *Everyday Nursing Ethics* (London: Macmillan).

Mental Capacity Act (2005), Great Britain (London: HMSO).

Mental Health Act (1983), Great Britain (London: HMSO).

Metcalfe A. and Burton, H. (2003), 'Postregistration genetics education provision for nurses, midwives and health visitors in the UK', *Journal of Advanced Nursing* 44(4) , pp. 350–9.

Midgeley, M. (1991), *Can't We Make Moral Judgements?* (Bristol: Bristol Press).

Mill, J. S. (1863), 'Utilitarianism', in Warnock, M. (ed.) (1962), *Utilitarianism* (London: Fontana).

Mill, J. S. (1859) 'On liberty', in Warnock, M. (ed.) (1962), *Utilitarianism* (London: Fontana).

Moskop, J. C. (1983), 'Rawlsian justice and a human right to health care', *The Journal of Medicine and Philosophy,* 8, pp. 329–38.

Mulhall, S. and Swift, A. (1992), *Liberals and Communitarians* (Oxford: Blackwell).

Nicholson, L. J. (1983), 'Women, morality and history', in Larrabee (ed.) (1993), pp. 87–101.

Noddings, N. (1984), *Caring: A Feminine Approach to Ethics and Moral Education* (Los Angeles: University of California Press).

Nordenfelt, L. (1995), *On the Nature Health* (Dordrech: Kluwer).

Nortvedt, P.(1996), *Sensitive Judgment, Nursing, Moral Philosophy, and an Ethics of Care* (Sats: Tano Aschehoug).

Nozick, R. (1974), *Anarchy, State and Utopia* (Oxford: Blackwell).

Nursing and Midwifery Council (2004), *The NMC Code of Professional Conduct; Standards for Conduct, Performance and Ethics* (London: NMC).

Nursing and Midwifery Council (2008), *The Code: Standards of Conduct, Performance and Ethics for Nurses and Midwives* (London: NMC).

O'Brien, A. J. and Golding C. G. (2003), 'Coercion in mental healthcare: the principle of least coercive care', *Journal of Psychiatric and Mental Health Nursing* 10, pp. 167–73.

Oderberg, D. S. (2000), *Moral Theory, a Non-Consequentialist Approach* (Oxford: Blackwell).

Ockleford, E., Berryman J., and Hsu, R. (2003), 'Do women understand pre-natal screening for fetal abnormality?' *British Journal of Midwifery*, July 2003, 11(7), pp. 445–9.

Okin, S. (1987), 'Justice and gender', *Philosophy and Public Affairs*, 16, pp. 42–72.

Paley, J. (2002), 'Virtues of autonomy: the Kantian ethics of care', *Nursing Philosophy* 3(2), pp. 133–43.

Plato, *The Republic* (trans) Lee, D. (1956) (Harmondsworth: Penguin).

Popkin, R. and Stroll, A. (1969), *Philosophy Made Simple* (London: Heinemann).

Public Concern at Work (available at: http://www.pcaw.co.uk./legislation/legi-lation.html) accessed 16/4/08.

Rachels, J. (1986), *The End of Life* (Oxford: Oxford University Press).

Rachels J. (1993), *The Elements of moral Philosophy* 2nd edn (New York: McGraw-Hill).

Raphael, D. D. (1981), *Moral Philosophy* (Oxford: Oxford University Press).

Raphael, D. D. (1990), *Problems of Political Philosophy*, 2nd edn (London: Macmillan).

Rawls, J. (1971), *A Theory of Justice* (Oxford: Oxford University Press).

Reinders, H. S. (2000), *The Future of the Disabled in Liberal Society* (Indiana: University of Notre Dame Press).

Robertson, G. (1993), 'Resuscitation and senility: a study of patients' opin-ions', *Journal of Medical Ethics* 19, pp. 104–7.

Rowson, R. (1990), *An Introduction to Ethics for Nurses* (London: Scutari Press).

Russell, B. (1912), *The Problems of Philosophy* (Oxford: Oxford University Press).

Ross, P. (1994), *De-Privatising Morality* (Aldershot: Avebury).

Schecter, W. P. (1992), 'Surgical care of the HIV-infected patient', *Cambridge Quarterly of Healthcare Ethics* 3, pp. 223–8.

Schon, D. A. (1987), *Educating the Reflective Practitioner* (San Francisco: Jossey-Bass).

Scott, P.A. (1995), 'Care, attention and imaginative identification in nursing practice', *Journal of Advanced Nursing* 21(6), 1196–200.

Scott, P. A. (2000), 'Emotion, moral perception and nursing practice', *Nursing Philosophy* 1(2), pp. 123–33.

Seedhouse, D. (1988), *Ethics the Heart of Health Care* (Chichester: John Wiley).

Seedhouse, D. (1998), *Ethics the Heart of Health Care* 2nd edn (Chichester: John Wiley).

Sellman, D. (2000), 'Alaisdair MacIntyre and the professional practice of nurs-ing', *Nursing Philosophy* 1(1), pp. 26–33.

Sheldon, S. and Wilkinson, S. (2004), 'Should selecting saviour siblings be banned?', *Journal of Medical Ethics* 30(6), pp. 533–7.

Silva, M.C. (1989), *Ethical Decisionmaking in Nursing Administration* (Norwalk, CT: Appleton and Lange).

Singer, P. (1979), *Practical Ethics* (Cambridge: Cambridge University Press).

Singer, P. (1993), *Practical Ethics*, 2nd edn (Cambridge: Cambridge University Press).

Singer, P. (ed.) (1986), *Applied Ethics* (Oxford: Oxford University Press).

Singer, P. (ed.) (1991), *A Companion to Ethics* (Oxford: Oxford University Press).

Sipes-Metzler, P. R. (1994), 'Oregon health plan: ration or reason?', *Journal of Medicine and Philosophy* 19, pp. 305–14.

Smart, J. J. C. and Williams, B. (1973), *Utilitarianism for and Against* (Oxford: Clarendon Press).

Tadd, V. (1991), 'Where are the whistleblowers?', *Nursing Times* 87 (1), pp. 42–4.

Thompson, I. E., Melia, K. M. and Boyd, K. M. (1988), *Nursing Ethics* (London: Churchill Livingstone).

Thompson, I. E., Melia, K. M. and Boyd, K. M. (2000), *Nursing Ethics*, 4th edn (London: Churchill Livingstone).

Tronto, J. (1987), 'Beyond gender difference', in Larrabee (ed.) (1993), pp. 240–57.

Tronto, J. (1993), *Moral Boundaries, a Political Argument for an Ethic of Care* (New York: Routledge).

UKCC (1984), *Code of Professional Conduct* (London: UKCC).

UKCC (1989), *Exercising Accountability* (London: UKCC).

UKCC (1992), *Code of Professional Conduct* (London: UKCC).

Viens, D. C. (1990), 'AIDS and ethics', *California Nurse* (November), pp. 8–12.

Voluntary Euthanasia Society (1992), *The Last Right: The Need for Voluntary Euthanasia* (London: VES)

Van Hooft, S. (1995), *Caring, an Essay in the Philosophy of Ethics* (Colorado: University Press of Colorado).

Verkerk, M. (2001), 'The care perspective and autonomy', *Medicine, Healthcare and Philosophy* 4, pp. 289–94.

Watson, J. (1985), *Nursing: Human Science and Human Care* (Norwalk: Appleton-Century-Crofts).

Wainwright, P. (1997), The Practice of Nursing, an Investigation from the Perspective of the Virtue Ethics of Alasdair Macintyre, Unpublished Doctoral Thesis, University of Wales, Swansea.

Westwood, G., Pickering, R., Latter, S., Lucassen, A., Little, P. and Temple, I. K. (2006), 'Feasibility and acceptability of providing nurse counsellor genetics clinics in primary care', *Journal of Advanced Nursing* 53(5), pp. 591–604.

Wilkinson, S. and Garrard, E. (2005), 'Passive euthanasia', *Journal of Medical Ethics* 31, pp. 64–8.

Williams, B. (1972), *Morality: an Introduction to Ethics* (Harmondsworth: Penguin).

Wilmot, S. (2000), 'Nurses and whistleblowing, the ethical issues', *Journal of Advanced Nursing* 32(5), pp. 1051–7.

Wolff, R. (1977), *Understanding Rawls* (Princeton: Princeton University Press).

Woods, S. and Edwards, S. D. (1989), 'Philosophy and health', *Journal of Advanced Nursing* 14, pp. 661–4.

Woods, S. (2007), *Death's Dominion, Ethics at the End of Life* (Buckingham: Open University Press).

Wright, S. (1993), 'What makes a person?', *Nursing Times* 89(21), pp. 42–5.

Yarling, R. R. and McElmurry, B. J. (1983), 'Rethinking the nurse's role in "do not resuscitate" orders', *Advances in Nursing Science* 5, pp. 1–12.

Index

abortion, 2
Agar, 183
acts and omissions, 83–6
Act Utilitarianism, 26–7, 38, 39, 40, 44–6
advocacy, 65
Alderson, P., 150, 153, 154, 157, 158, 176, 177, 179, 195
Alzheimer's Society, 135–6
American Nurses Association (ANA), 4
Aristotle, 41, 44, 87, 153
Armstrong, A.E., 41
autonomy, 26, 57–63, 98–100

Baier, A., 153
Beauchamp, T. L. and Childress, J. F., 18–29, 47–9, 57, 59, 63, 66, 68–74, 80, 81, 85, 86, 87, 100, 110–21, 130, 134, 138, 148, 172, 202, 205–6, 214, 215, 217, 218, 220
beneficence, 27, 74–81
Benjamin, M. and Curtis, J., 4, 57, 63, 110–17, 120–1, 125, 143, 198
Benner, P. and Wrubel, J., 149
Bentham, J., 29
Berghmans, R. and Widderhoven, G., 125
Bloch, S. and Heyd, D., 124–7
Blum, L., 162, 164, 177
Bowden, P., 169
Brabeck, M., 154
BRCA1/2 gene, 200
British Medical Association, 108

Buchanan, A. E. and Brock, D. W., 61, 73, 189, 195
Burnard, P. and Chapman, C. M., 4

Camus, A., 125
Capuzzi, C. and Garland, M., 143
Card, C., 169
care as 'moral orientation', 174–6
caring claim, 152, 161, 170, 172
categorical imperative, 37–9
Chadwick, R. and Tadd, W., 4
Chamberlain, W., 96–7
competence, 63–73
confidentiality rule, 23–4
Clouser, D. and Gert, B., 148
Cox, P., 184
Curtin, L. and Flaherty, M. J., 163, 210

Daniels, N., 137
'David' case, 79–80
Deontology, 34–41
de Raeve, 22
Dickenson, D., 129
dignity, 103–4
Dock, L., 45
do not resuscitate (DNR) decisions, 108–9
Dooley, D. and McCarthy, J., 204, 210
Downs Syndrome, 184–96

emotions claim, 152, 165
ethical disorientation, 11
expressivist objection, 188

Faulder, C., 65
fidelity rule, 24–6, 21, 43
Friedman, M., 155

Gastmans, C., 174
Gilligan, C., 149–70
Gillon, R., 57, 75, 99, 129, 131, 135
Glover, J., 84, 126
Gough, E., 81, 121

Hare, R. M., 50, 160
Harris, J., 28, 126, 141
Harris, C., 136
Harris, L., 136
Herceptin, 136
Hewitt, J., 125
hierarchy-web distinction, 157–9,
    167–8
HIV, 213–14
Human Tissue Act (2004), 23
Hunt, G., 210
Huntington's Disease, 197–9
Hursthouse, R., 47
Hussey, T., 7

Jehovah's Witnesses, 81, 121–2
Johnstone, M. J., 214
Justice, 27, 86–98, 99, 171
justice-claim, 152, 164

Kant, I., 34–41
Kohlberg, L., 149–51
Kuhse, H. and Singer, P., 84
Kymlicka, W., 97, 153, 155

life plan, 59, 62, 190, 191, 219–20
Little, M., 174
Loach, E., 191
Loehy, E. H., 109
Lutzen, K., 58

Marquis, D., 194
Mason, J. K. and
    McCall Smith, R. A., 61
Melia, K., 63
Mental Capacity Act (2005), 100
Mental Health Act (1983), 52, 58,
    66, 83
metaethics, 5
Midgeley, M., 167
Mill, J. S., 29, 57, 93

mixed-sex wards, 1
moral awareness, 7–8
moral judgements, 18–19
morally relevant characteristics, 77–82
moral perception, 7–8
moral rules, 20–6
moral sensitivity, 7–8
moral subjectivism, 167

needs/wants distinction, 138
NMC Code, 6, 45, 51, 54, 61, 74,
    75, 80, 81–3, 90–2, 98, 101–4,
    130, 145, 198, 208–11,
    217, 219
Noddings, N., 149, 171, 178
nonmaleficence, 27, 80–3
Nordenfelt, L., 50
Nortvedt, P., 174
Nozick, R., 94–8, 99, 145,
    195, 196
nurses 'station', 216–17

objective-subjective distinction, 156–7,
    166–7
O'Brien, A.J. and Golding, G.C., 63
Ochleford, E., Berryman, J. and
    Hsu, R., 190
Oderberg, D., 85
Oregon Plan, 143–4

Paley, J., 41
paternalism, 110–27, 198
Patient's Charter, The, 40, 108, 110,
    132, 137
person/human being distinction, 28
persons, respect for, 28
Pink, G., 204
Plato, 144, 153
privileged-view claim, 152, 161, 163
public-domestic distinction, 155,
    165–6
Public Interest disclosure
    Act (1998), 205
privacy rule, 22–3

Rachels, J., 38
Raphael, D. D., 5
Rawls, J., 93–8, 99, 142, 145, 153, 196
reflective equilibrium, 48
Reinders, H.S., 191, 192
Rescher, N., 131

resource allocation
  desert-based, 139–41
  needs-based, 136–9
  rights-based, 132–6
  utility-based, 131–2
rights, positive and negative, 134
Robertson, G., 109
Rowson, R., 107
Royal College of Nursing, 108

Schecter, W. P., 216
Scott, P.A., 11, 178
Seedhouse, D., 3, 17, 50, 60, 138,
  160, 208
self-project, 59
Sellman, D., 173
Sheldon, S. and Wilkinson, S., 183
Singer, P., 3, 60, 85, 90, 154,
  162, 170
suicide, 123–7

Tadd, W., 210
Thompson, I. E., Melia, K. M. and
  Boyd, K. M., 4
Tronto, J., 162, 169–74
trust, 22
truth-telling, 107–8

UKCC Code of Conduct, 4, 74,
  203, 204
UK-Plan, 144–5
UK resuscitation council, 108
uniqueness claim, 151–2,
  160–1
Universalizability, 160–1
Utilitarianism, 4, 29–33
utility, principle of, 30

van Hooft, S., 62, 169
veracity rule, 21
virtue ethics, 41–7
Voluntary Euthanasia
  Society, 124

Wainwright, P., 173
Westwood, G., 184
Wilkinson, S. and Garrard, E., 85
Williams, B., 33
Wilmot, S., 204
withdrawing and withholding
  treatment, 85
Woods, S., 5, 61

Yarling, R. R. and
  McElmurry, B. J., 109